The Gentle Art of YOGA

for healthy, joyful ageing

What is the body?
That shadow of your love
That somehow contains the whole universe.

– Rumi

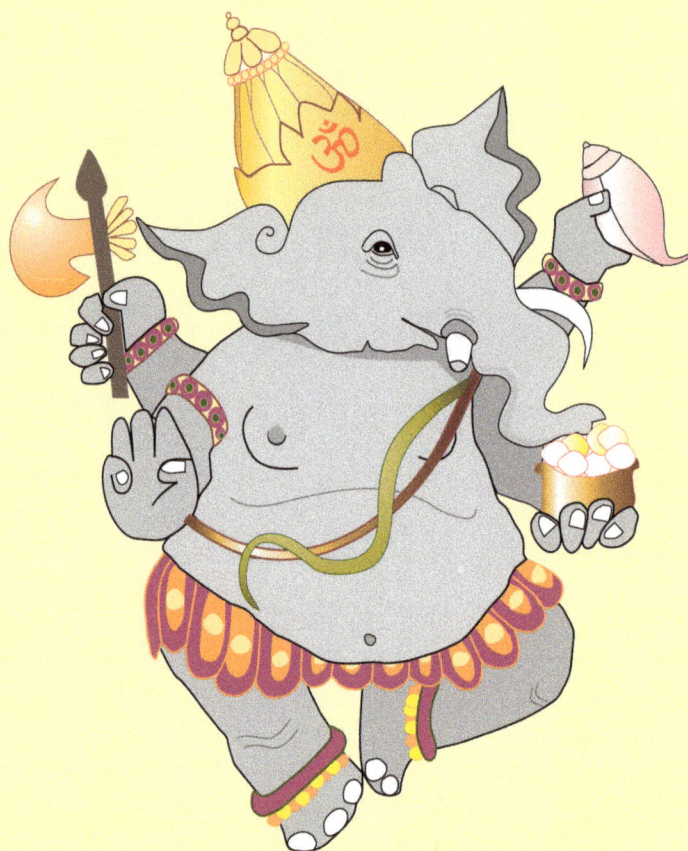

Ganesha

The Remover of Obstacles

Lord Ganesha is invoked for auspicious beginnings,
so it is appropriate that he appears at the beginning of this book
in the fervent hope that the reader will enjoy the contents.

Illustration © Sharon Kirchner

The Gentle Art of
YOGA

for healthy, joyful ageing

Sharon Kirchner

For Octavia and Temperance

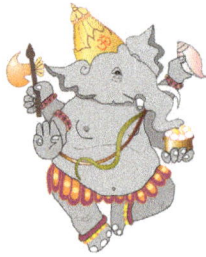

Copyright © 2017 Estate of Sharon D Kirchner

Published by Artemis Press, Leura NSW 2780, Australia

ISBN-10: 0-646-97718-0

ISBN-13: 978-0-646-97718-8

Email: gentleartofyoga@tutanota.com

Book design: Sharon Kirchner

Production and cover: Louise Bennett (Chintanshuddhi)

Photography: Michael Cox

Contents

Foreword

This book is published posthumously. My mother Sharon was diagnosed with pancreatic cancer just as the manuscript was completed and she did not get the chance to see the book through to publication before she died on 9 April 2017.

With the help of some of Sharon's friends, relatives and former students, the book has now been published as a memorial to her and so that her vast knowledge and experience of the discipline of yoga is not completely lost to the world.

I saw firsthand Mum's evolution from student to teacher of yoga over the course of her life. I remember sitting at the back of the hall at Bondi Public School doing my primary school homework while she did yoga classes in the 1970s. Over time, this led to formal yoga studies and then accreditation with the International Yoga Teachers Association. Mum's interests were not limited to yoga. She was knowledgeable in all of the Vedas, including studying Jyotish with Hart de Fouw.

Mum's knowledge was grounded not only in her formal and informal learning, but also in 15 years of experience teaching yoga in Leura, in the Blue Mountains to the west of Sydney. Her classes were notable for their diversity and Mum's inclusive attitude meant that people of all ages, ability and physical fitness were able to benefit from her approach.

It was only after she died that I became fully aware of how important her classes were in the lives of so many people. Typical of the messages I received from her students include the following:

I will love Sharon forever for the way she inspired and guided me through my yoga practice.

I was diagnosed with a debilitating chronic disease in 2002 and it was recommended that I go to Sharon's yoga classes. I had never practised yoga before and from the very first class I realised that it was going to be very special.

These weekly classes and Sharon's friendship and understanding have helped to keep me going through all my challenges...

During all the years I never made excuses for not attending classes. It was my number one priority as I realised the health benefits to my life.

I have missed the classes terribly over the last year but have been inspired by Sharon's positive attitude and perseverance.

She has left me with a wonderful gift of the tools I need to continue my yoga practice at home. I will always hear her voice encouraging and guiding me.

Another message I received was typical of the responses to the news of her death:

I thought the world of your mum... I was always struck by her inner and outer beauty and grace. She was a truly special person and I feel blessed to have known her.

It is my hope that through the publication of this book, many more people will benefit from Mum's knowledge, experience, creativity and inspiration.

Mum's ashes are scattered along the Prince Henry Cliff Walk between Olympian Rock and Elysian Rock. If you enjoy this book and happen to find yourself in Leura, I hope you can visit that place and think of her.

I would like to thank the following people for their assistance and also generously donating their time in making this publication possible: Louise Bennett (Chintanshuddhi), Susan Hili, Leah Hili, and Michael Cox.

In loving memory,

Stephen Kirchner

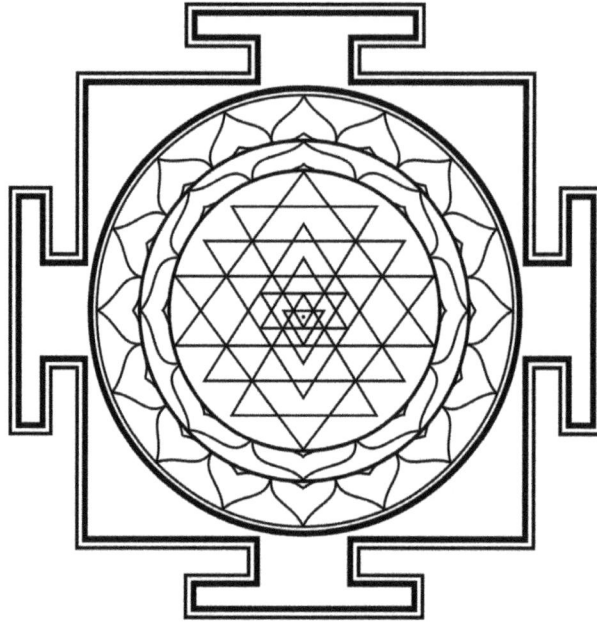

Sri Yantra

One of the most auspicious, important and powerful of the Yantras,
the Sri Yantra is the sound vibration of the cosmic Aum.

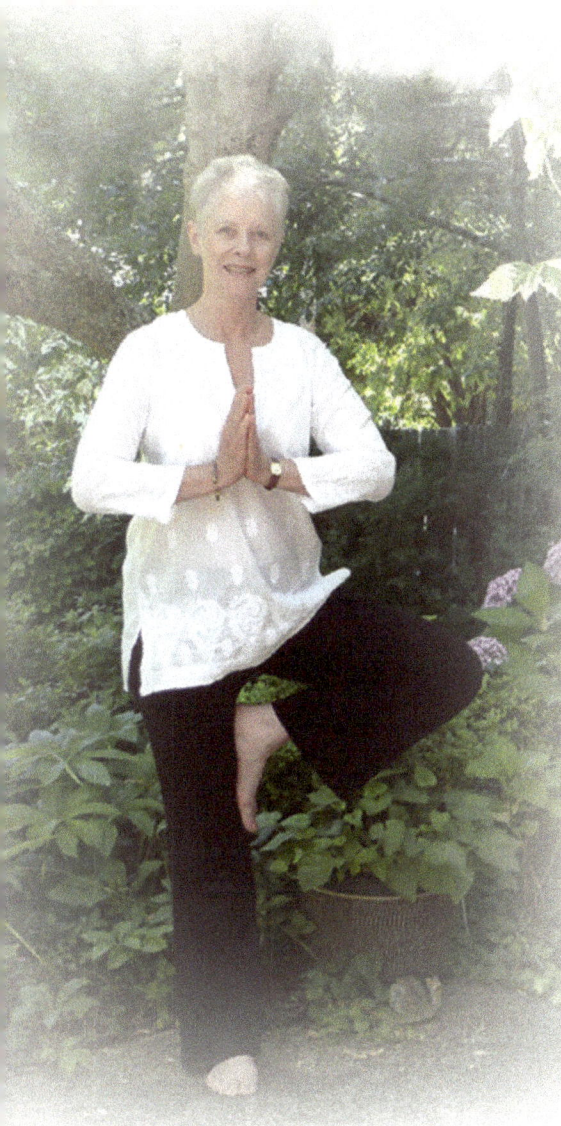

Namaste,

Often when I mention I teach yoga, a common response from mature age people is "I couldn't possibly do yoga, I'm too stiff and inflexible." All the more reason to do yoga, is my response.

In fact, yoga is the perfect practice for ageing bodies. Its strength lies not only in maintaining supple joints, but it enhances a general sense of wellbeing and confidence – qualities that are particularly important as the body ages. It can help to lower blood pressure, build strength and help you feel younger, vibrant and more alive.

Through the gentle practices of yoga, you will become more aware of your body and how it works. The postures, breath work and meditation techniques will help your body and mind to work as one, leaving you feeling relaxed, calm and centred, and more able to cope with the pressures of life.

Maybe you are concerned about your ability to deal with the physical aspects of yoga?

With help from mature age yogis from my classes (sixty years plus in age), I have endeavoured to show how you can modify the positions if the full posture remains out of your reach. Also, modifications can help ease you into yoga until your body is strong and supple enough to do the full practice.

All you need to practise yoga is a quiet space and your mat. It's that simple.

Yoga has been such a deeply rewarding experience in my life, and if you are not practising yoga already, then I hope this book encourages you to give it a go. It will change your life in limitless ways – all of them for the better.

Sharon

The meaning of NAMASTE

I honour that place in you of love, of light, of truth, of peace.

And if you are within that place in you, and I am within that place in me,

Then there is only one of us.

Yoga Overview

There are as many different types of yoga as there can be many different pathways to the top of a mountain, but all of them have the same view and goal – union. That is what yoga means: 'union' or 'yoke.' The union of body, mind and breath, the union of individual consciousness with universal consciousness, bringing mind, body and spirit to a state of balance and harmony.

There are many different branches of yoga and so it is important to choose the path that best suits your nature. There are many different limbs on the 'tree of yoga' such as Jnana Yoga (the yoga of knowledge), Bhakti Yoga (devotional yoga), Japa Yoga (sound vibration), Karma Yoga (selfless service) and Raja Yoga (meditative practices). There is also a form of yoga that deals with the energy centres of the body called Kundalini Yoga, as well as Tantra Yoga and many other disciplines.

Hatha Yoga, a branch of yoga that emphasises physical and mental control of the body, as well as cleansing practices, has become a term to loosely describe most of the yoga taught in classes in the West. However, there are various forms of this discipline and classes can vary widely, depending on which tradition the teacher comes from. Therefore, it is important to find a class and teacher that best suits your individual needs.

To fully experience yoga, your class needs to encompass not only asanas (postures), but pranayama (breath control), pratyahara (sense withdrawal/relaxation) and dharana/dhyana (meditation).

Yoga is involved in every aspect of life, so once you begin the yogic journey there are many interesting and rewarding paths to follow. Ayurveda is also a yogic discipline which focuses on health and wellbeing. Yoga has an amazing history based on ancient philosophy and psychology which is as relevant today as it was centuries ago. The ancient yogic texts and scriptures are a fascinating study. The *Bhagavad Gita*, written over 2,500 years ago, being an excellent example.

There is no limit to the amazing journey that is yoga.

The Yoga of Patanjali

All yoga teachers and most yoga practitioners are familiar with Patanjali's *Yoga Sutras*. Patanjali was a sage who lived around 200 BCE and was responsible for the first written text on yoga: the *Yoga Sutras*. *Sutras* are wise sayings or aphorisms that were originally handed down by word of mouth.

Patanjali's *Yoga Sutras* is still regarded as the premier text on yoga at its very heart. They describe a sequence of eight stages or steps which, if followed, will lead to self-realisation (samadhi) – the goal of yoga.

Patanjali's Yoga is also known as Raja Yoga or Ashtanga Yoga.

The eight limbs or aspects of Raja Yoga are:

Yamas: Restraints, universal ethical disciplines

Niyamas: Observances, rules of conduct applying to individual discipline

Asana: Physical postures

Pranayama: Vital energy or breath control

Pratyahara: Sense withdrawal

Dharana: Concentration

Dhyana: Meditation

Samadhi: Illuminated consciousness

The sections of this book fall into the eight categories of Patanjali's Yoga Sutras, as the Sutras give an accessible pathway to understanding the discipline that is yoga.

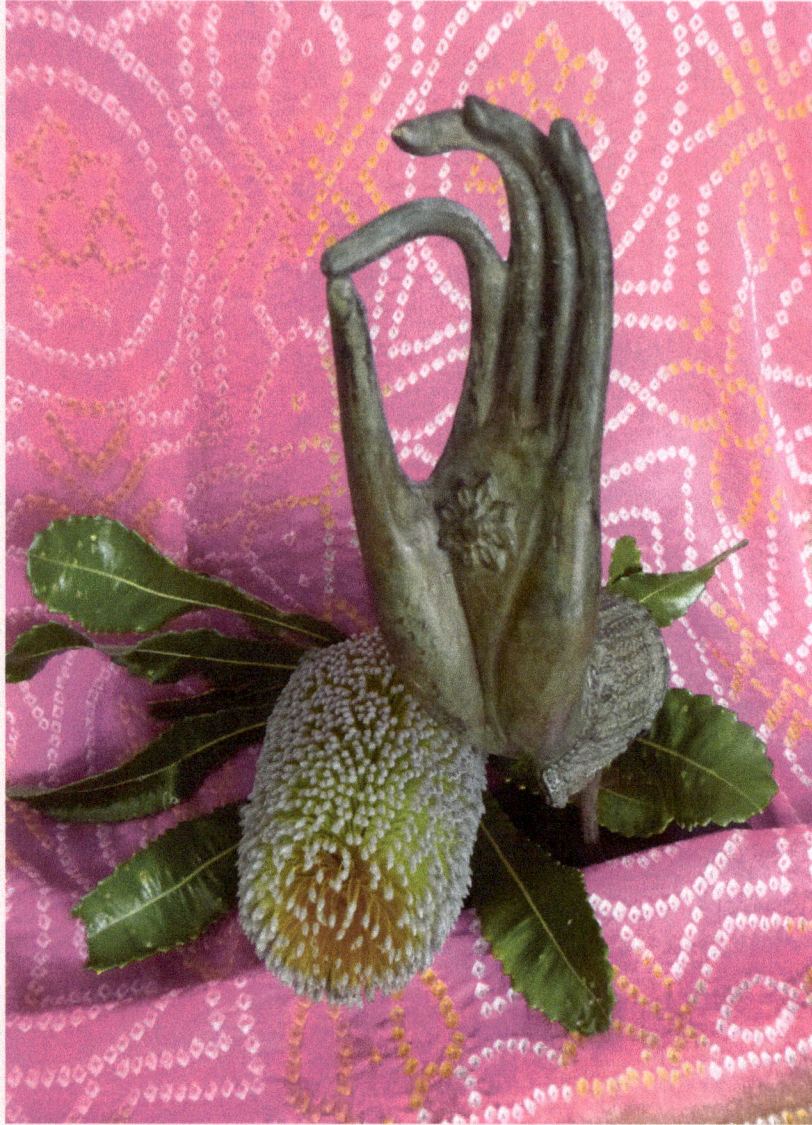

Yamas and Niyamas

*Ethical Standards, Self-Discipline
and Spiritual Observances*

Yamas and Niyamas

According to Patanjali's *Yoga Sutras*, to attain the peak of yoga experience the whole human being should be balanced and in harmony. This is achieved not only through asana, pranayama and meditation, but by observing certain disciplines and ethical standards. Traditionally, the Yamas and Niyamas were considered preparatory practices to be mastered before the other yoga practices were embarked upon. They are still considered the framework for all yoga practice, but are ideals to aspire for – a constant work in progress. The following offers a short description of these guidelines:

Yamas deal with one's ethical standards and sense of integrity. They are universal in nature.

❖ *Ahimsa*: Non-violence – to avoid harm to all living creatures by thought, word or deed. Violence and anger come from fear, weakness and ignorance.

❖ *Satya*: Truth – this means truthfulness in thought, word and deed. Not limited to speech alone 'being true to yourself' is another aspect of truthfulness.

❖ *Asteya*: Non-stealing – this not only refers to material things, but to stealing knowledge or the wisdom of another, to steal another's self-confidence or even their joy.

❖ *Brahmacharya*: All body energies and creative forces should be conserved and used wisely.

❖ *Aparigraha*: Non-covertousness – another facet of non-stealing. To be free from hoarding is *aparigraha*. We should not hoard or collect things that others may also need.

Niyamas deal with self-discipline and spiritual observances and are more individual in nature.

❖ *Saucha*: Purity and cleanliness – this includes cleansing the mind of disturbing emotions, cleansing the intellect of impure thoughts, purity in the food we eat, cleanliness of the place we live in and where we practise yoga.

❖ *Santosa*: Contentment – you need to be content to concentrate and to maintain control of the mind, otherwise energy is wasted in worry and fear.

❖ *Tapas*: Austerity and a burning effort under all circumstances to achieve a definite goal in life. The whole science of character-building may be regarded as a practice of *tapas*. Weaknesses are overcome, inner strength and willpower are developed.

❖ *Svadhyaya*: Study or education of the self. Education is the drawing out the best that is within a person.

❖ *Isvara Pranidhana*: Self-surrender – surrender to a higher power, letting go of the ego.

In Summary

Not to harm, lie, steal, over-indulge, or desire more than you actually need;
instead be content, pure, self-disciplined, studious and devoted.

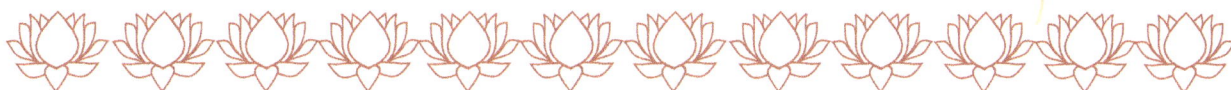

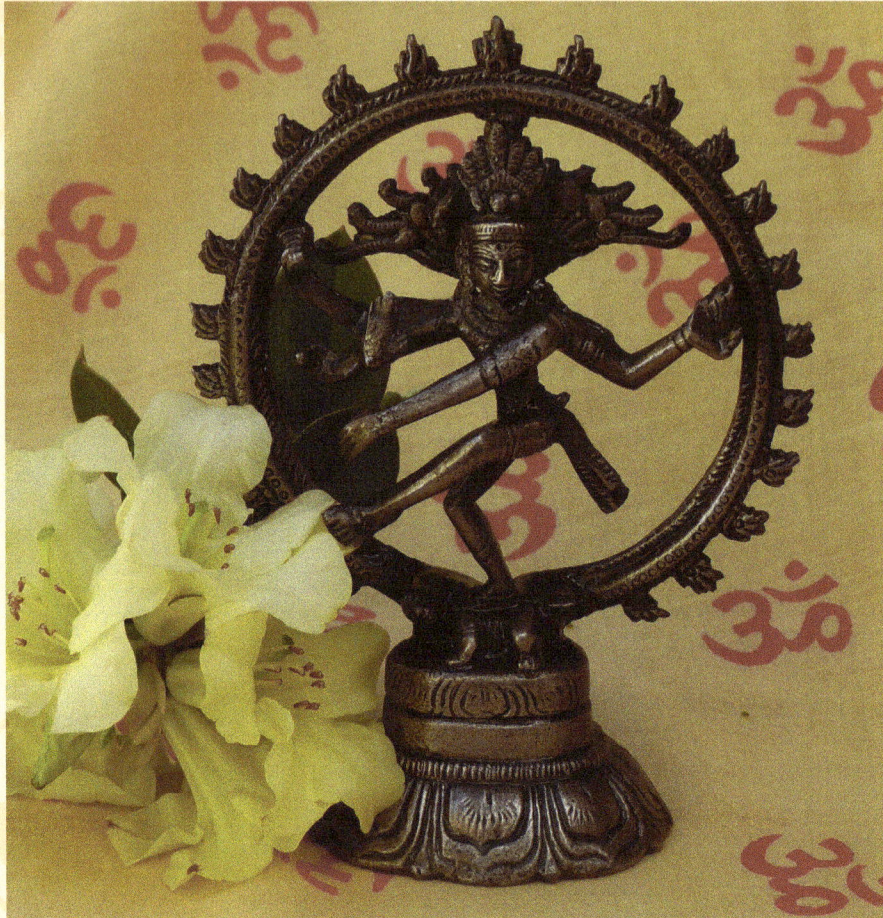

Asana

Postures

The practice of asanas purges the body of its impurities,
bringing strength, firmness, calmness and clarity of mind.

– *BKS Iyengar*

Asana Overview

The first yama (discipline) is ahimsa, harmlessness, and this must be your first priority when practising yoga. The approach to asana is with an attitude of kindness and acceptance of your limitations, to remain relaxed, focused and work with the breath. Bring an open curiousty to the practice, with mind and body working as one.

If you feel discomfort in your body or if the body starts to shake, you need to slowly come out of the pose and modify your approach. Take note of the cautions that are listed at the bottom of the asana demonstration pages.

Modifications

There is a strong emphasis in this book on modifications. When we first come to yoga, especially in advanced years, the body may not be flexible enough to perform the full asana. Until the body is flexible and strong, it is important to modify the pose. Modifications are shown and described with this symbol throughout the book. ❀

Counterposes

If a strong forward bend, back bend, side stretch, inversion or twist is held for any length of time, it is important to counterpose immediately afterwards so that the spine can find its neutral position once again and the muscles of the body can relax before moving on to the next asana. Generally the counterpose is held for half the length of the original pose. Counterposes will be shown where advisable in the demonstration pages.

Limbering

It is important to do simple stretching and work with the joints before moving into your asana sequence. Some limbering suggestions appear on page 58.

Breathing

Diaphragmatic (abdominal) breathing is generally practised through-out the asana session. Unless otherwise stated, inhalation and exhalation is done through the nose. Usually it is an inhalation at the commencement of the pose when extending limbs away from the body, and an exhalation to release into the pose. Once in the asana, relax and breathe freely.

Physical fitness

If you are unsure of your fitness level to practise yoga, or if you are beginning yoga at a mature age, then first consult your doctor.

You can practise yoga at any age, whether it be 10, 20, 40, 60 or 80, because the practices begin gradually and are simple enough to exercise the different parts of the entire body. It is not necessary to practise advanced yoga like standing on your head or performing intricate contortions. Asana is a practice through which you attain awareness of the body, release tension and stress from different joints and muscles, and come to a state of relaxation in which you are physically comfortable in whatever you do.

– Swami Niranjanananda Saraswati

ASANA CONTENTS

Standing Postures (Page 10)

- Tadasana – *Mountain Pose*
- Utkatasana – *Chair Pose*
- Nitambasana – *Hip Stretch Pose*
- Dwikonasana – *Double Angle Pose*
- Trikonasana – *Triangle Pose*
- Trikonasana Variation
- Padottanasana – *Intense Forward Stretch*
- Konasana – *Side Angle Pose*
- Virabhadrasana I – *Warrior 1 Pose*
- Virabhadrasana II – *Warrior 2 Pose*
- Sirsangusthana – *Head to Toe Pose*
- Padahastasana – *Hands to Feet Pose*
- Uvasvastikasana – *Squat Pose*
- Urvasana – *Thigh Pose*
- Pristha Vakrasana – *Back Arch Pose*
- Kati Chakrasana – *Waist Rotating Pose*

Balancing Postures (Page 20)

- Natarajasana – *Dancer Pose*
- Vriksasana – *Tree Pose*
- Garudasana – *Eagle Pose*
- Tuladandasana – *Flying Balance Pose*
- Virabhadrasana III – *Warrior 3 Pose*
- Navasana – *Boat Pose*
- Merudandasana – *Spinal Balance Pose*
- Chandrasana – *Crescent Moon Pose*
- Natarajasana – *Lord Shiva's Dance*
- Utthita Hasta Padangusthasana – *Hand to Big Toe*
- Flamingo Pose

Kneeling Postures (Page 27)

- Vajrasana – *Thunderbolt Pose*
- Pranatasana – *Pose of the Child*
- Simhasana – *Lion Pose*
- Anjangyasana – *Lunge Pose*

- Ardha Ustrasana – *Half Camel Pose*
- Ustrasana – *Camel Pose*
- Parighasana – *Gate Pose*
- Sasamgasana – *Hare Pose*
- Threading the Needle
- Vyaghrasana – *Tiger Pose*
- Chatuspadasana – *Quadruped Pose*
- Chest Opening Laterel Stretch
- Marijariasana – *Cat Pose*
- Gomukhasana – *Face of a Cow Pose*

Seated Postures (Page 36)

- Dandasana – *Rod Pose*
- Purvottanasana – *Backward Plank Pose*
- Paschimottanasana – *Forward Stretch Pose*
- Janu Sirshasana – *Head to Knee Pose*
- Easy Seated Spinal Twist
- Matsyendrasana – *Lord of the Fish Pose*

Supine/Prone Postures (Page 40)

- Shavasana – *Corpse Pose*
- Advasaṅa – *Prone Corpse Pose*
- Dhanurasana – *Bow Pose*
- Sarpasana – *Snake Pose*
- Sphinx
- Bhujangasana – *Cobra Pose*
- Urdhva Mukha Svanasana – *Upward Facing Dog Pose*
- Ardha Salabhasana – *Half Locust Pose*
- Salabhasana – *Locust Pose*
- Salabhasana Variation – *Flying Locust Pose*
- Setu Bandhasana – *Bridge Pose*
- Supta Pawanmuktasana – *Leg Lock Pose*
- Pelvic Lifting
- Supta Udarakarshanasana – *Sleeping Adominal Stretch Pose*

Yoga postures are quite often known by more than one name depending on which tradition they have come from. I have chosen the name that I feel is most commonly used.

This is by no means the full range of yoga postures. The ones chosen are those commonly practised in most yoga traditions and are well within the reach of mature age yoga practitioners.

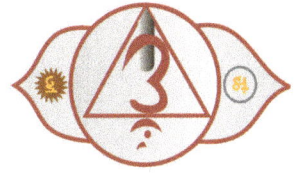

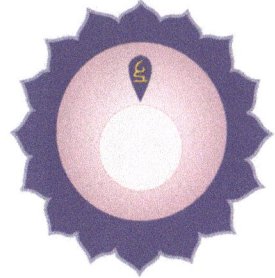

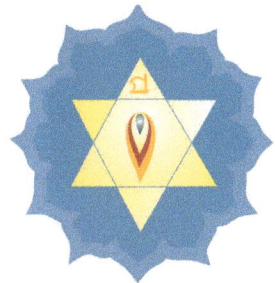

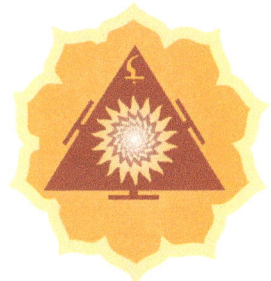

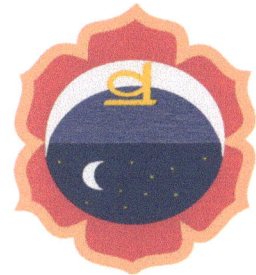

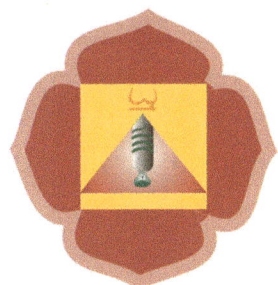

Tadasana – *Mountain Pose*

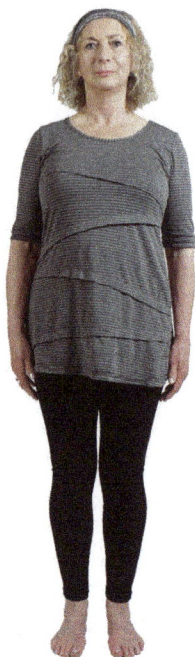

Utkatasana – *Chair Pose*

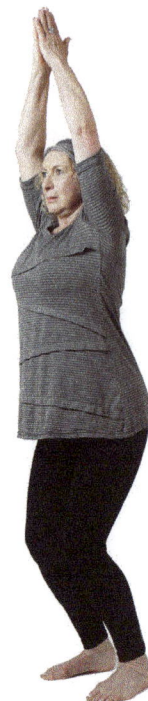

This posture is the starting position for many of the standing asanas.

Stand with the feet slightly apart, with the inner edges parallel and with the weight evenly distributed over both feet.

Gently rock backwards and forwards on the feet and make the rocking less and less until you find your natural centre of gravity.

Soften the knees and gently activate the core muscles (draw the navel back towards the spine). Lift the sternum.

Roll the shoulders forward, lift them high and draw them back behind you, and then gently release the arms.

Relax the shoulders and let the arms hang loosely beside the body with the palms facing inwards. Have the chin tucked in a little.

The *drishti* (gaze) is forward.

Feel that you are inhaling up through the feet, lifting and lengthening through your body. Be aware of the breath and every part of your body.

Benefits: In this pose the body is in perfect alignment.

Tip: This is a good asana to practice while standing in the check-out queue at the supermarket.

Begin in Tadasana. Step the feet hip-width apart. Inhale and raise the arms out to the sides and up over the head, arms parallel and palms of the hands facing each other. The arms stay alongside the ears throughout the practice.

Exhale, bend the knees and lower the body as if to sit in a chair. The upper body can have a slight tilt forward. (Can also be done with a straight back).

Hold the pose for as long as is comfortable, breathing freely.

To release, inhale and straighten the legs, exhale and lower the arms.

Benefits: Works the toes, and strengthens the ankles, calves, knees and thighs.

Cautions: Do not practise this pose if you have severe knee conditions.

The posture is mastered and perfect when all effort is relaxed and the mind is absorbed in the Infinite.

– Patanjali's Yoga Sutras

Nitambasana – *Hip Stretch Pose*

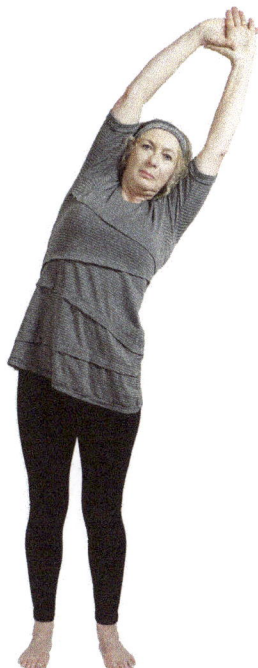

This asana is relatively simple but prepares the body for all the side bending asanas.

Stand in Tadasana with feet together and facing forward. Inhale, raise the arms over the head, palms together or overlapping thumbs, arms alongside the ears, and ears well away from the shoulders.

Exhale, extend to the right side, making sure the left shoulder does not roll forward. Keep the arms straight. Extend through the spine and lengthen the back of the neck.

Maintain your position and inhale.

As you exhale, take the side stretch a little further. Exhaling deeper into the stretch can be repeated several times until you have reached your limit.

Inhale to come out of the pose slowly.

Repeat to the other side.

Modification: ✹ To modify, step the feet a little wider apart.

Benefits: The stretch to the side includes the spine, ribcage, arms, shoulder joints, waist and hips. This lateral stretch will help keep your back supple and strong.

Cautions: Go gently if you have lower back issues.

You are as young as your spine!

Dwikonasana – *Double Angle Pose*

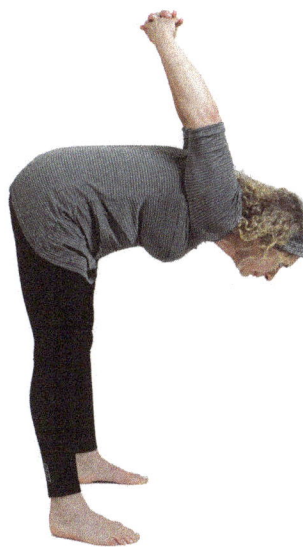

Stand in Tadasana. Step the feet a little more than hip-width apart.

Interlock the hands behind the back, inhale and stretch up, lengthening through the spine.

Exhale, fold forward from the hips while simultaneously raising the arms behind the back as high as possible without straining.

Keep looking forward so that the face is parallel to the floor to keep the spine in alignment. Focus on the breath. The arms in this position act as levers to accentuate the stretch to the shoulders and chest. Remain in this position a short time, breathing freely. To release, bring the arms to rest on the buttocks, bend the knees and on an inhalation, raise slowly to the upright position.

Modification: ✹ Bring hands to the hips and then fold forward, keeping the back parallel to the floor.

Counterpose:

Benefits: Strengthens muscles in the back and works on flexibility of the shoulder joints. Opens the chest and strengthens the neck muscles.

Cautions: Not appropriate if you have high blood pressure or any shoulder joint conditions. Modify.

Trikonasana – *Triangle Pose*

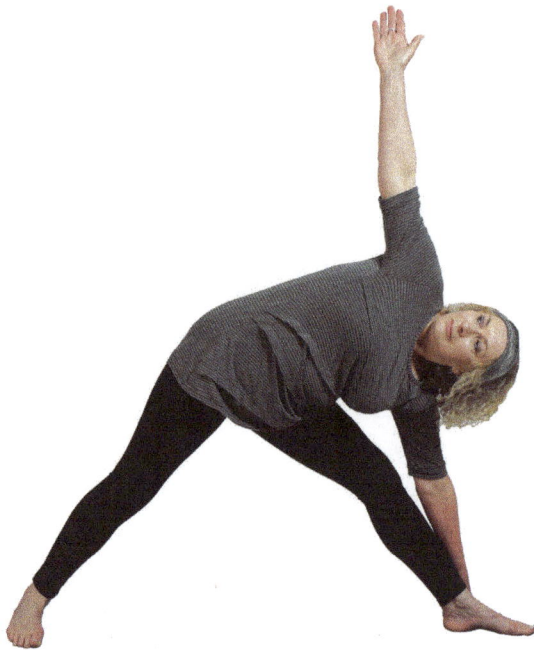

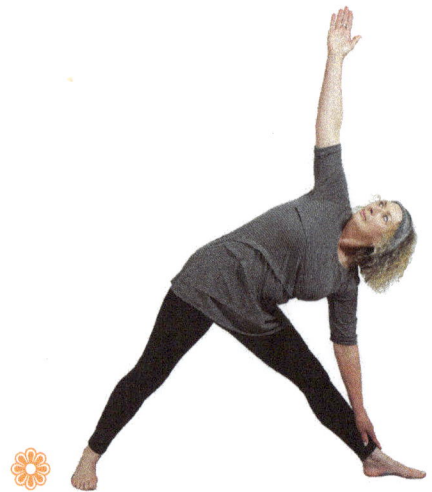

Face forward or look up at hand.
Bend knee if needed.

Stand in Tadasana. Step the right foot approximately one metre from the left and turn the right foot out 90⁰ to the left foot. The right heel is centred with the left instep.

Inhale, float arms to shoulder height.

Exhale, moving from the hips, glide to the right side.

Bring the right hand to the floor on the outer side of the right ankle. Place the left hand behind the waist to open the chest and avoid the left shoulder rolling forward. Then take the left hand to the shoulder, raise elbow and extend arm upwards, palm facing forward. If there are no neck problems, turn to look up to the right hand.

To release, inhale and raise the body to the upright position, arms at shoulder height. Exhale, lower the arms and step feet back together. Breathe freely.

Repeat to the other side.

Modification: ✴ Bring the right hand to rest on the ankle, shin or knee, if the floor is out of reach. If you have neck problems, instead of looking up to the hand, look straight ahead.

Counterpose: This 🧍 or 🧍

Benefits: Tones, strengthens and stretches muscles in the entire body.

Cautions: If you have any lower back conditions be very careful with this pose and definitely only do the modified version. Care should be taken with shoulders and neck as well. Modify as needed.

It is through the alignment of the body that I discovered the alignment of my mind, self, and intelligence.

Asanas maintain the strength and health of the body, without which little progress can be made. Asanas keep the body in harmony with nature.

– B.K.S. Iyengar

Trikonasana Variation

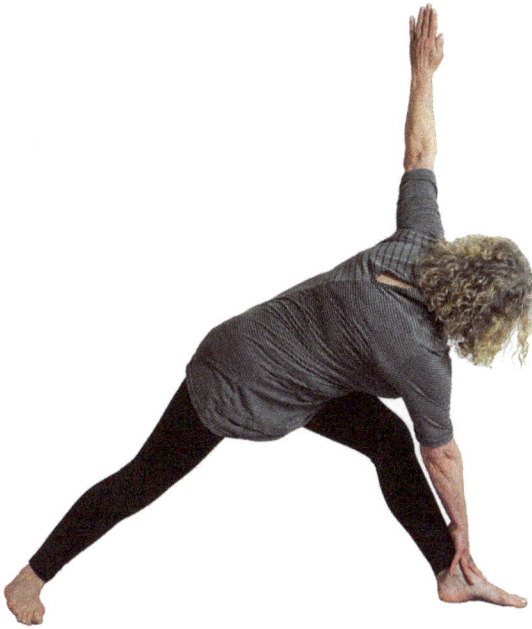

Stand in Tadasana with the feet approximately 1 metre apart with the feet slightly angled out to the side. Place the hands on the hips.

Inhale, lift up tall through the body and fold forward to make a flat back. Exhale and take the right hand to the left foot and curl the fingers around the side of the foot if possible. When steady, inhale and raise the left arm to vertical so that both arms form a straight line. Look up to the left hand. Breathe freely and hold for as long as is comfortable.

Inhale, bring both hands to the hips while still folded forward with a straight back. Exhale and repeat to the other side.

Modification: ✹ Bend the knees if the hamstrings feel overstretched. Place hand on the shin if you cannot reach the foot.

Counterpose:

Benefits: Excellent lateral and hamstring stretch. This pose improves digestion, activates intestinal peristalsis and strengthens the pelvic area.

Cautions: Not appropriate if you have back conditions or high blood pressure. Modify.

Padottanasana – *Intense Forward Stretch*

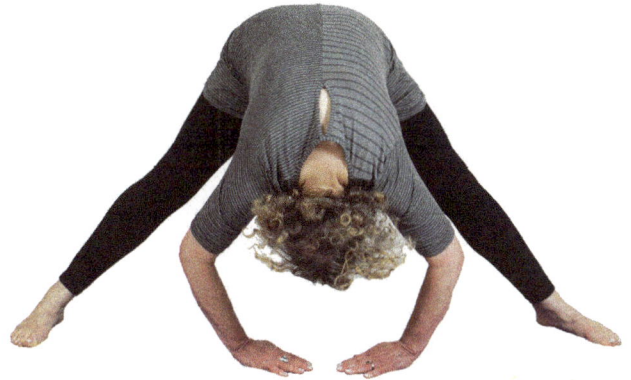

Stand in Tadasana.

Inhale, step the feet wide apart with the feet parallel or turned slightly outwards.

Place the hands on the hips. Inhaling, lengthen through the spine and firm the abdomen.

Exhale, fold forward from the hips, keeping the torso in a straight line and hold for a few moments. Inhale, then exhale, draw in the abdomen and lift the buttocks high. Place the hands on the floor, fingertips in line with the toes, or pointing inwards if more comfortable. Bend the elbows and bring the head towards the floor, as far as possible.

Modification: ✹ Keep the hands on the hip and have the torso parallel to the floor.

Counterpose:

Benefits: Stretches the legs, spine, hips and tones the abdominal organs.

Cautions: Not appropriate for high blood pressure, eye or back problems. For these conditions, do the modification only.

Parshvakonasana – *Side Angle Pose*

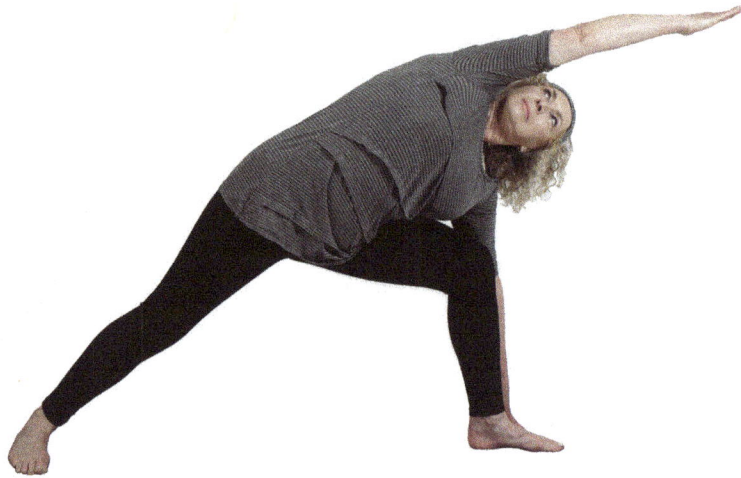

Stand in Tadasana. Place the hands on the hips.

Inhale, and on exhalation take a wide step to the side. The right foot is at a 90° angle to the left, and the heel aligns with the instep of the left foot. The left foot points straight ahead or slightly inwards. The hips and chest face forward.

Stage 1: Inhale, raise the arms to shoulder height with the palms turned down. Exhale, bend the right knee until it is directly over the ankle, the thigh parallel to the floor. Inhale and lift the body out of the pelvic girdle, exhale and glide to the right, resting the right forearm on the right thigh while turning the left palm up and raising the left arm parallel to the side of the head. Press the feet firmly into the floor, and lengthen from the left heel through to the left fingertips.

Stage 2: Release the right arm from the thigh and place the hand on the floor at the outside of the right foot. Keep the right arm and leg together. Rotate rib cage and abdomen and lift the chest away from the pelvis. Keep the neck long, look straight ahead, or turn the head to look up if there are no neck problems.

Modifications: ❀ Stage 1 only.

Counterpose: This or

Benefits: Develops strength and flexibility, increases mobility in hip joints, strengthens the quadriceps and all muscles of the legs and pelvis. A strong lateral stretch for the entire body.

Cautions: Be careful with this pose if you have back problems. Do modification only.

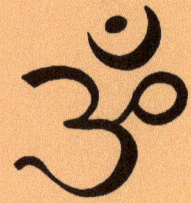

The symbol of Aum

Mantra is a pure sound vibration which frees the mind from its limitations. Aum is the core mantra, the vibration of creation manifested as sound.

The world of matter in which we live is composed of different qualities and densities of sound vibrations.

Sound originates as pure silence and descends into denser and denser frequencies until matter is formed. Still residing at the heart of matter is the vibrational experience of Aum.

All matter is vibrating and the sound of that vibration is Aum.

– Swami Niranjanananda (Satyananda Yoga)

Virabhadrasana I – *Warrior I Pose*

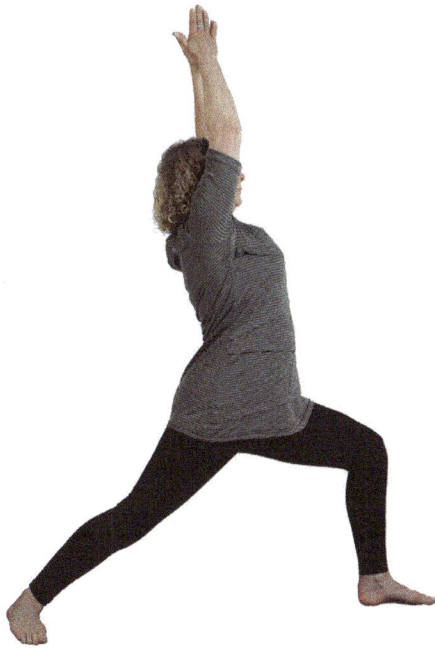

Stand in Tadasana at the top of the mat, feet hip-width apart and toes pointing forward.

Inhale, then exhale and take a large step behind with the left leg. Hips are facing forward, the left foot slightly angled to the side. Inhale and raise the arms overhead, vertical and parallel, palms facing.

Lift and lengthen through the body.

Exhale, bend the right knee to a lunge, forming a right angle, the knee directly above the ankle. Look straight ahead with the chin slightly tucked in.

Hold for as long as is comfortable, breathing freely.

To release, inhale and straighten the knee, exhale and lower the arms. Step the left foot forward to the right foot.

Repeat to the other side.

Modification: ✿ For lower back problems, lean slightly forward so as not to put pressure on the lower vertebrae. Place hands on the hips if there are shoulder problems.

Counterpose:

Benefits: Improves concentration and balance, and works the toes, ankles, knees, hips, shoulders and spine.

Cautions: Can be a problem for the lumber spine, knees, shoulders, and for untreated high blood pressure.

Virabhadrasana II – *Warrior 2 Pose*

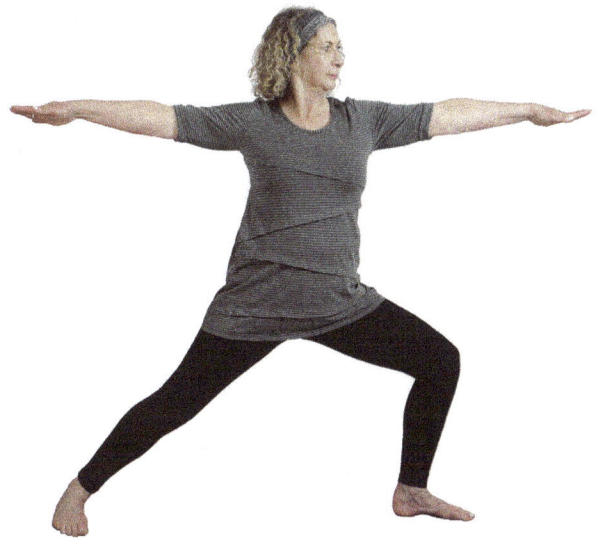

Stand in Tadasana. Step the right foot out to the side, the foot at a 90⁰ angle to the left foot and the heel aligned with the instep of the left foot. The left foot faces slightly inwards. The hips and trunk of the body remain facing forward throughout the pose. Maintain equal weight on both feet.

Inhale, lift the spine and float arms up to shoulder height, palms facing downwards. Exhale, bend the right knee so that the right thigh is parallel to the floor and the shin is perpendicular to the floor.

Then turn the head to look at the middle finger of the right hand. Focus on the breath and remain in the posture as long as it is comfortable. Repeat to the other side.

To release, inhale, straighten right leg. Exhale, bring the feet together and lower the arms.

Modification: ✿ Do several times to each side, holding for short periods until the body is strong enough to hold for any length of time.

Counterpose:

Benefits: Strengthens the whole body. Excellent weight bearing asana and builds core strength.

Cautions: Avoid if there are severe knee problems.

Sirsangusthasana – *Head to Toe Pose*

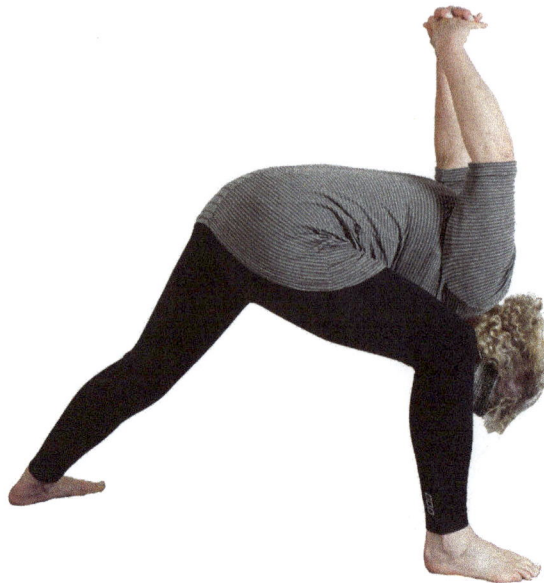

Advanced version: Stand at the top of the mat, feet hip-width apart. Hands are interlocked behind, resting on the buttocks.

Inhale then exhale and step the left leg behind, foot turned outwards about 45^0. Make sure the hips are facing forward. Inhale, lift up through the body and exhale to come into a lunge, the right shin parallel to the floor with the knee above the ankle.

Inhale, lengthen through the spine, then exhale and fold forward from the hips bringing the head towards the floor on the inside of the right ankle. (For advanced practitioners the crown of head may touch the floor).

Raise the arms straight back and up in line with the shoulder joints. Elbows may be slightly bent if it's impossible to straighten the arms.

To release, bring the hands to rest on the buttocks, and raise the head to the knee. Place weight on the right leg and push yourself upright through this leg.

Return to Tadasana.

Repeat to the other side.

Counterpose:

Benefits: Strengthens the whole body. Works the back, legs, shoulder joints and abdominal muscles.

Cautions: Not appropriate for untreated blood pressure, or problems with the heart, shoulder joints or eyes.

Modified: ❀ Stand at the front of the mat, with feet hip-width apart. Take the arms behind and hold opposite elbows.

Inhale, then exhale and step the left leg behind, foot turned outwards about 45^0. Make sure the hips are facing forward. Inhale, lift up through the body, exhale and come into a lunge, the right shin parallel to the floor with the knee above the ankle.

Inhale, lengthen through the spine and exhale, fold forward from the hips to where the chest is in line with the knee. Rest the shoulder on the knee.

To release, place the weight on the right leg and push yourself upright through this leg.

Return to Tadasana.

Repeat to the other side.

Benefits: Same as the advanced pose but to a lesser degree.

Cautions: Not appropriate for untreated blood pressure, or problems with the heart, shoulder joints, or eyes.

Padahastasana – *Hands to Feet Pose* (Dynamic Version)

Padahastasana – *Modification*

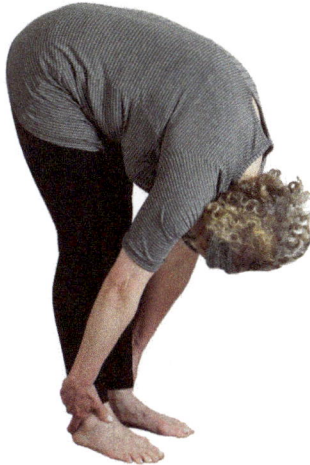

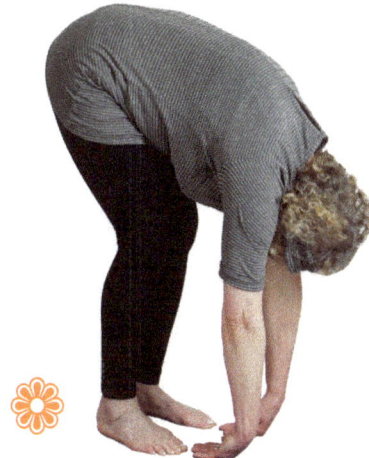

Stand in Tadasana. Lengthen the spine, and distribute the weight of the body evenly over both feet.

Inhale, raise both arms overhead, palms facing forward. Lean backwards slightly to lengthen through the body. Exhale, draw in the abdomen and fold forward from the hips, torso parallel to the floor. Inhale, extend further forward.

Exhale, lower from the hip joints. Place hands on either side of the feet, fingers in line with the toes. If that's not possible then hold the lower legs or ankles.

If it is still within your comfort zone, bring the forehead to the straight knees but do not overstretch the hamstrings by forcing this movement. Hold for a few seconds to begin with and let your spine passively release and let the head hang heavy.

To release, place hands on the hip joints and point the elbows up to the ceiling. Keep the head in line with the spine, bend the knees, inhale and lift the torso to upright.

Modification: ✳ As per adjoining column.

Counterpose:

Benefits: Tones digestive organs, spine and spinal nerves. Increases blood flow to the head. Increases vitality.

Cautions: Not appropriate for blood pressure issues, eye problems, lower back and knee problems.

Stand in Tadasana. Lengthen the spine, and distribute the weight of the body evenly over both feet.

Inhale, bring the chin to the chest, and with bent knees, slowly roll the body forward, relaxing the shoulders forward and letting the arms go limp. Imagine there are no bones or muscles in the body – just dangling forward. Let gravity do the forward stretch for you. Stay in this position if it feels like the body has reached its limit.

Provided you are not forcing or straining the body, place the fingers under the toes.

To release, place hands on the hip joints and point the elbows up to the ceiling. Keep the head in line with the spine, bend the knees, inhale and lift the torso to upright.

Counterpose:

Benefits: Tones digestive organs, spine and spinal nerves. Increases blood flow to the head. Increases vitality.

Cautions: Not appropriate for blood pressure issues, eye problems, lower back and knee problems. For these conditions, only do the first stage of this modified version.

Avasvastikasana – *Squat Pose*

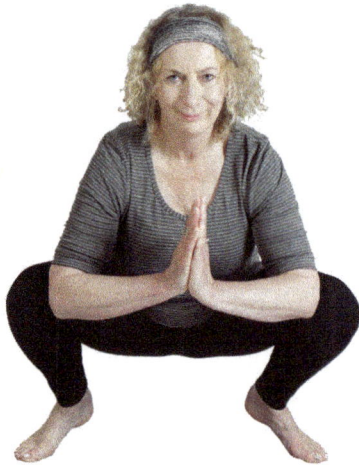

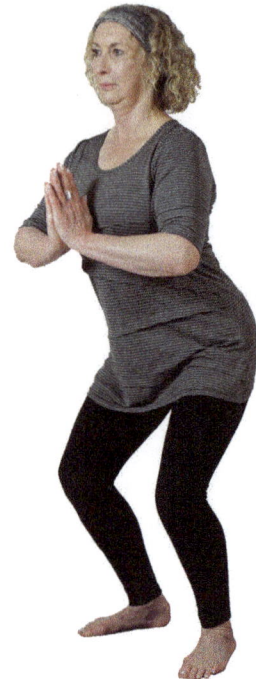

Stand in Tadasana. Place the hands in Anjali Mudra (prayer position).

Feet are a little more than hip-width apart and angled out slightly to the sides.

Inhale, then exhale and lower into a squat, making sure that the knees are at the same angle as the feet. The upper arms push against the inner thighs, keeping the knees in alignment over the feet. Heels remain on the floor.

Hold for as long as is comfortable, breathing freely, then slowly return to Tadasana.

Modification: ✺ If your heels are lifted off the floor, then place a folded blanket under the heels for support.

Benefits: Stretches the hips, thighs, calves, ankles, toes.

Cautions: Absolutely *not appropriate* for people with knee problems. Do Urvasana in the adjoining column for a similar result with less strain on the knees. Can also be difficult for those with weak hips and ankles.

Urvasana – *Thigh Pose*

Stand in Tadasana. Place hands in Anjali Mudra (prayer position).

Stand with feet hip-width apart and angled out slightly to the sides.

Inhale, then exhale and bend the knees and tilt the body slightly forward keeping the knees at the same angle as the feet. Keep the head, neck and spine aligned. Keep the weight of the body on the heels.

Hold for as long as is comfortable, breathing freely, then inhale and return to Tadasana.

Benefits: Stretches the hips, thighs, calves, ankles, toes.

Cautions: Still not appropriate for *severe* knee conditions but not as stressful as Avasvastikasana. Use discretion and if the pose causes discomfort, then discontinue the practice.

*When you convince your mind of its
accomplishing power, you can do anything.*

– Paramahansa Yogananda

Pristha Vakrasana – *Back Arch Pose*

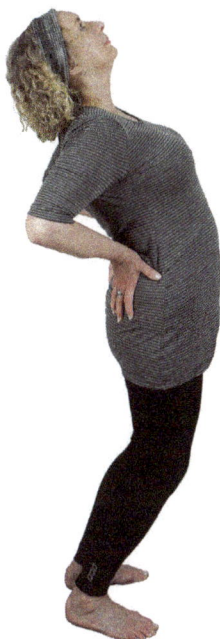

Stand in Tadasana.

Place the hands on the lower back, placing the heels of the hands either side of spine at the waist. Spread the fingers, pointing them downwards. This protects the lower back.

Inhale and lengthen through the body. This is important so that on arching back you allow room for the vertebrae to stretch. Exhale and gently arch backwards. Keep the face relaxed.

Inhale and raise the body to upright. Return to Tadasana.

Benefits: This works on flexibility of the spinal column and also benefits the adrenal glands.

Tip: This pose can be used for counterposing standing forward bends. Also a great relief for the back after gardening.

Kati Chakrasana – *Waist Rotating Pose*

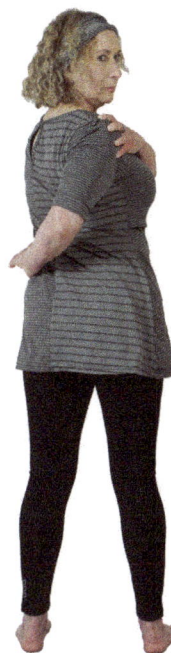

Stand in Tadasana.

Step the feet hip-width apart with the toes turned slightly inwards. This helps to avoid undue strain on the knees when twisting.

Inhale and raise the arms to the sides at shoulder height, exhale and slowly twist the body to the right side, the left hand pressing gently on the right shoulder and the right hand is wrapped around the left side of the waist.

Keep the back of the neck long and have a sense that the body is revolving around a fixed point at the top of the spine. Hold the breath for a few seconds, then inhale and return to the starting position.

Exhale and repeat to the other side. Do several rounds from side to side, holding for a few counts on each side.

Benefits: Strengthens and tones the waist, spine, back and hips.

*Keep knocking, and the joy inside
will eventually open a window
and look to see who's there.*

– Rumi

Natarajasana – *Dancer Pose (Modified)*

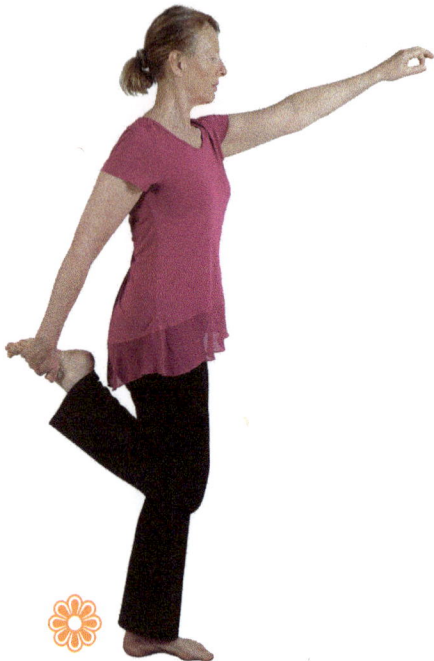

Natarajasana – *Dancer Pose*

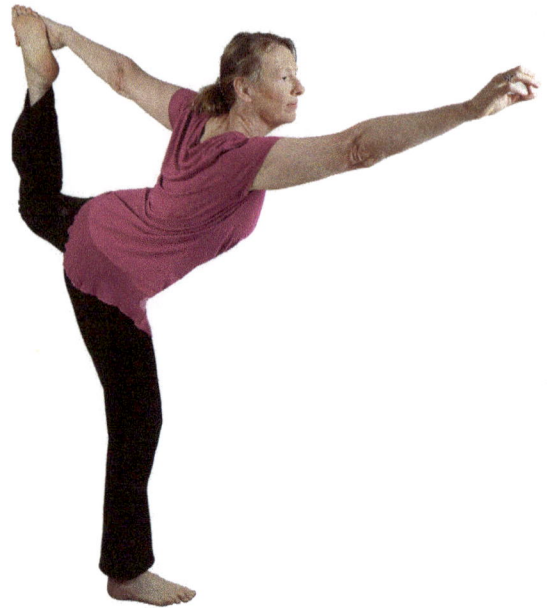

Modification: ✤ The modification of this pose is perfect for balance and coordination training. In this asana, we can transition from the modified version to the full version of Natarajasana in adjoining column.

Stand in Tadasana. Close your eyes and centre your mind for a few minutes.

Transfer your weight to the left leg and raise the right knee to the chest. Slide the right hand down to the ankle – hold the ankle firmly and point the knee towards the floor and bring the right foot towards the buttocks.

Once balanced, inhale and raise the free arm in front, slightly elevated, and adopt a hand mudra by joining the tips of the index finger and thumb.

Note: If you have difficulty staying balanced while you lift your leg, then stand sideways to a wall and touch the wall to steady yourself. When you feel secure, let go of the wall and slowly raise the other arm.

If you have difficulty holding on to the ankle or foot, then hold on to the bottom of your trouser leg until your flexibility improves.

Benefits: Improves concentration and strengthens the legs.

To do the full pose given here, continue on from the modification (left).

Keep the back lengthened and stretch from the left heel through your whole body right through to the fingertips.

Fold the right leg behind you, activate the leg muscles and move the heel away from the buttocks. Start to tilt forward a little.

Keep the pelvis and chest aligned to the front.

Note: You can also continue to tilt forward until the trunk and right thigh are parallel to the floor.

Breathe freely in the pose and then repeat for the same amount of time to the other side.

Benefits: Improves concentration and strengthens the legs, making them more supple. Also works the shoulders. A wonderful quadricep stretch.

Cautions: Go gently if lower back problems exist.

Vriksasana – *Tree Pose*

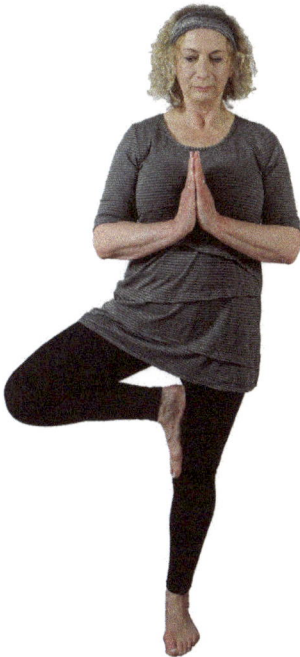

Stand in Tadasana. Close your eyes and centre your mind for a few minutes.

Open your eyes and focus your gaze on a fixed point (drishti) in front of you at eye level. Bend one leg, hold the ankle and place the sole of the foot high on the inner thigh of the other leg. Keep the knee turned out to the side, opening up the hip joint.

When you are steady, place the hands in prayer pose and stay in this pose, breathing freely, or to extend further you can inhale and raise the arms overhead, palms together, arms alongside the ears. Keep distance between the ears and the shoulders. Breathe freely.

Hold the pose steady and when it's time to release, lower the hands to the sides and the foot to the floor.

Repeat to the other side.

Modification: ✿ Place one foot on top of the other or on the calf of the standing leg. Palms are placed together at the heart space in prayer pose.

Benefits: Improves concentration and strengthens the legs, ankles and foot muscles.

Garudasana – *Eagle Pose*

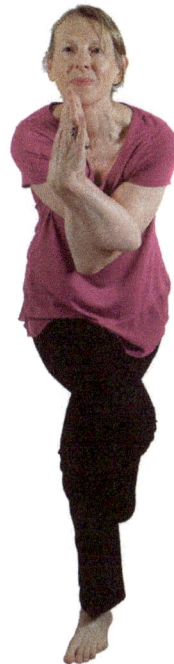

Stand in Tadasana. Close your eyes and centre your mind for a few minutes.

Open your eyes, inhale and raise the arms out to the sides at shoulder height. Exhale and fold the right arm over the left above the elbows, then wrap the lower arms around each other, ending with palms together, thumbs towards the face.

Slightly bend the right knee, and on an inhalation, cross the left leg over the right leg above the knee and tuck the foot behind the right calf.

Hold for as long as is comfortable.

To release, inhale and bring the left foot to the floor and unwrap the arms.

Repeat to the other side.

Modification: ✿ Place one foot on top of the other to maintain balance.

Benefits: Works the ankles, knees and hips. This pose also strengthens the leg muscles and opens the back, releasing stiffness in the shoulders. Relieves sciatica.

There is only one teacher – life.

– Author unknown

Tuladandasana – *Flying Balance Pose*

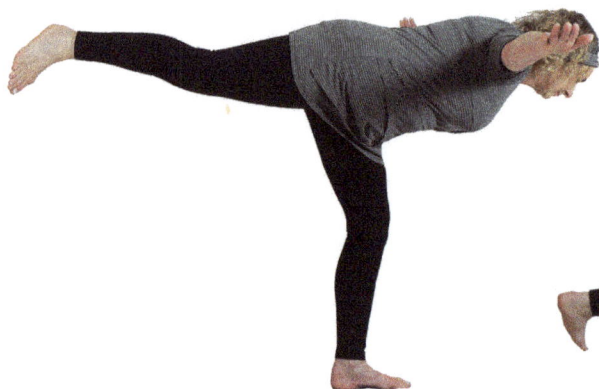

Virabhadrasana III – *Warrior 3 Pose*

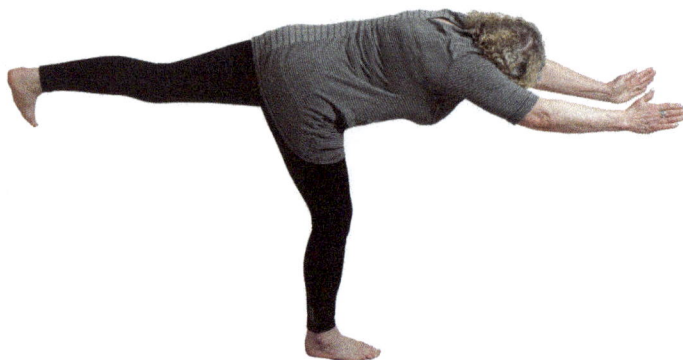

Stand in Tadasana. Close your eyes and centre your mind for a few minutes.

Inhale, lift the arms to the side to shoulder height with the palms facing towards the floor. Step forward with the right leg and transfer the weight of the body to the right leg.

Exhale, fold forward from the hips, raising the left leg straight behind you. The toes can point either back behind you or flexed to point to the floor.

Make sure the hips stay square to the floor. Imagine the body in a straight line from the head, through the torso to the foot.

Hold the posture for as long as is comfortable, breathing freely.

To release, inhale and raise the torso as the left leg lowers to the floor.

Repeat to the other side.

Benefits: Improves concentration and strengthens the legs and back muscles.

Cautions: Do not hyper-extend the support leg – keep it soft.

Stand in Tadasana at the top of your mat, feet hip-width apart. Close your eyes and centre your mind for a few minutes.

Inhale, then exhale and step the left leg behind. Make sure the hips are facing forward. Inhale, raise the arms overhead, vertical and parallel. Exhale and transfer the weight of the body to the right leg. Tilt forward until the body and the left leg are parallel to the floor.

Hold for as long as is comfortable, breathing freely.

To release, inhale and lower the left leg to the floor and the body to upright.

Repeat to the other side.

Benefits: Improves concentration and strengthens the legs and back muscles.

Cautions: Do not hyperextend the support leg. Can be an issue for lower back problems.

The source of unhappiness lies in ignorance;
Knowledge alone sets us free.

– Yogatattva Upanishad

Navasana – *Boat Pose*

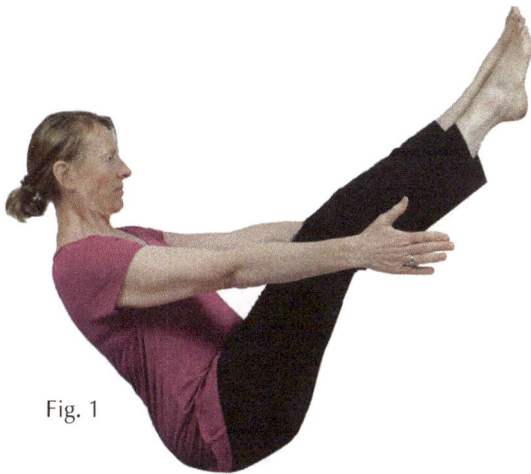
Fig. 1

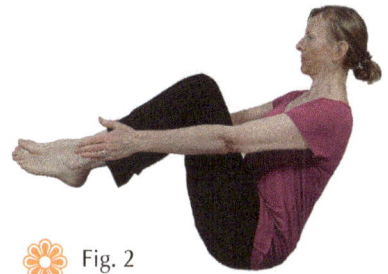
🌸 Fig. 2

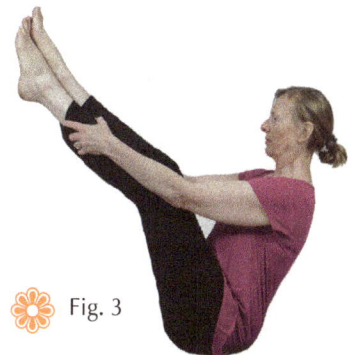
🌸 Fig. 3

Start in Dandasana with a straight back.

Draw the knees to the chest and tilt back slightly. In doing this, make sure the back doesn't hunch up.

Inhale, press back into your hands, and straighten the legs to a 45⁰ angle to form a V shape with the body. Exhale, raise the arms parallel each side of the knees with the palms facing each other. Tip the chin slightly towards the sternum. Balance on the buttocks (Fig. 1).

It is important to keep the spine as straight as possible, and not slump, as this puts pressure on your spine and not on your abdominal muscles.

Breathe freely and stay in the pose as long as it feels comfortable to do so. Gradually increase the time you stay in the pose to strengthen the abdominal muscles. Release the legs with an exhalation and relax.

Modifications: 🌸 Shorten the levers by bending the legs (Fig. 2) or by holding the legs (Fig. 3). It is best to practise the modifications until you are strong enough to hold the pose.

Counterpose:

Benefits: Strengthens the upper and lower abdominal muscles and benefits the back, spine and legs. Increases the ability to concentrate and balance.

Cautions: Do not practise this pose if you have back issues or have recently had an operation.

Yoga is far from simply being physical exercise, rather it is an aid to establishing a new way of life which embraces both inner and outer realities. However this way of life is an experience which cannot be understood intellectually and will only become living knowledge through practice and experience.

– Swami Satyananda Saraswati

Merudandasana –
Spinal Balance Pose

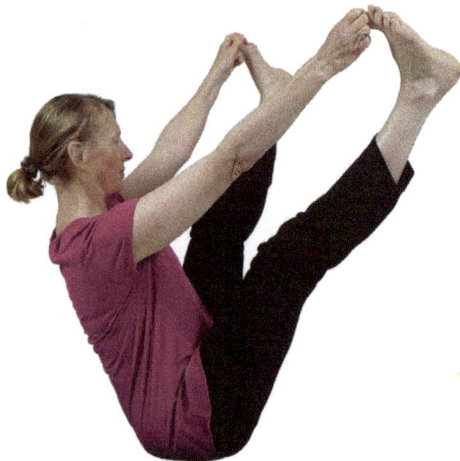

Ardha Chandrasana –
Crescent Moon Pose

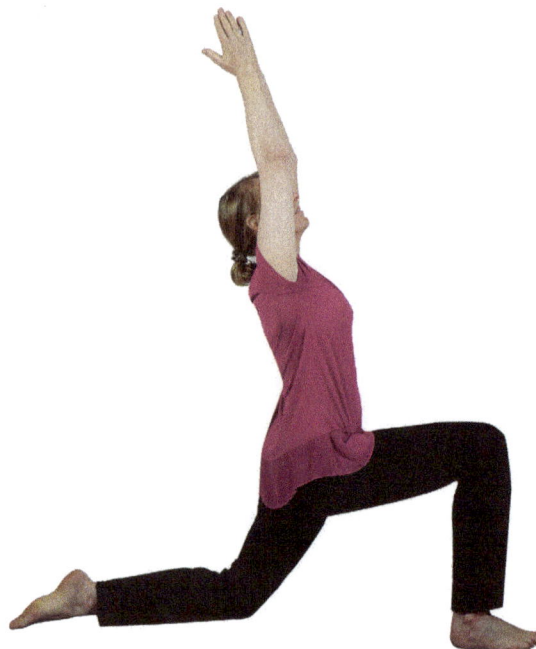

Start by sitting in Dandasana.

Bend the knees and bring the souls of the feet together. Place the thumb and forefingers around the big toes. Inhale, tilt slightly backwards and raise the legs wide apart, straightening the legs as much as possible. Keep the back straight, not slumping in the middle.

Balance on the buttocks while maintaining a straight spine.

Modifications: ✽ If you cannot straighten the legs, move the hands from the feet down to the ankles.

Counterpose:

Benefits: Strengthens and brings flexibility to the spine, hips and legs, and works the abdominal muscles. Increases the ability to concentrate and balance.

Cautions: Care should be taken if there are lower back problems.

Start by placing both knees on the floor.

Inhale, then exhale and lunge the right leg forward, taking care to form a 90^0 angle (to avoid straining the knee).

The left knee remains touching the floor.

Place both fingertips on the floor beside the right foot, in line with the toes.

Balance the body in this position for a moment.

Then inhale, raise both arms above the head and bring the palms together.

Lean back slightly to form a crescent moon curve with the trunk, and lift the head to look upwards.

Benefits: Strengthens the legs, hips and spine. Improves balance and concentration.

Cautions: This pose can be a problem for weak ankles and lower back issues, and for stiffness in the shoulders.

Note: This pose is also used in the sequence of Chandra Namaskara.

*If you think you can, or if you think you can't,
either way your're right.*

– Henry Ford

Natarajasana – *Lord Shiva's Dance*

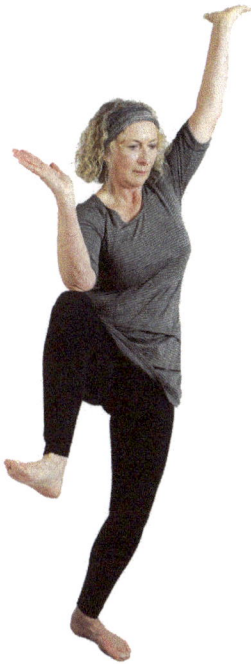

Utthita Hasta Padangusthasana – *Hand to Big Toe Pose*

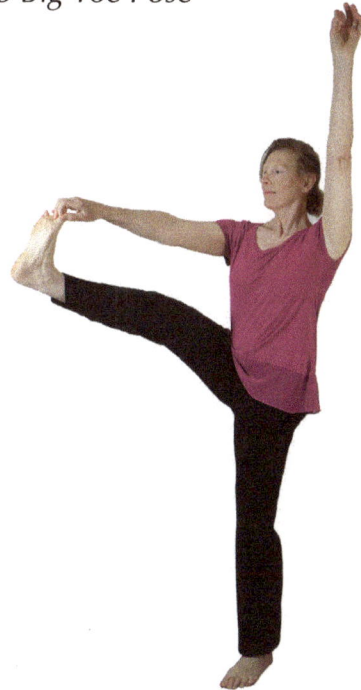

There are several versions of Natarajasana but this one I enjoy the most!

Stand in Tadasana.

Relax the body and focus the mind. Balance on your left leg and extend your left arm alongside your head, palm facing inwards and hand angled out to the side.

Bend your right leg, lifting it as high as possible off the floor and rotate your right inner thigh and calf outwards, flexing the foot.

Bend the right arm and place the elbow on the right knee. The palm faces upwards and angles out to the side.

Breathe freely, holding as long as possible on each side.

Benefits: This asana helps to balance the nervous system, and strengthens the legs, hips and spine. It gives a good lateral stretch to the body and improves balance and concentration .

Cautions: Can be a problem for weak ankles.

Stand in Tadasana.

Relax the body and focus your mind.

Bend the right leg and bring the knee as close as possible to the chest. Slide the right hand down the inside of the thigh and take hold of the right big toe.

Slowly try to straighten the right leg. To help you to balance, focus your gaze on a fixed point (drishti). When you feel steady, raise the left arm to vertical, elbow alongside the ear, and bring the tips of the index finger and thumb together to form a hand mudra.

Benefits: This asana helps to balance the nervous system, and strengthens the legs, hips and spine. It improves balance and concentration.

Cautions: Can be a problem for weak ankles and lower back issues .

Whatever affects one directly affects us all indirectly. I can never be what I ought to be until you are what you ought to be. This is the interrelated structure of reality.

– Martin Luther King

Flamingo Pose

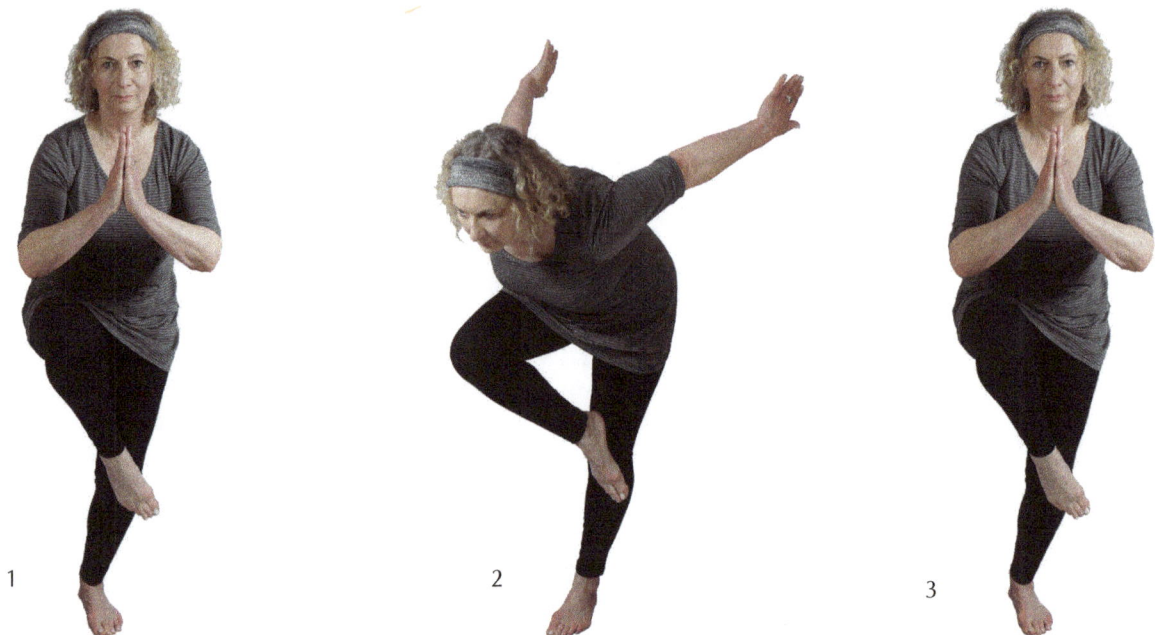

1   2   3

Thank you, Amoona Metcalfe, for this interesting balancing pose.

Stand in Tadasana.

Position 1: Inhale, then exhale and bend both knees into a half squat and place the right foot on top of the left knee. Place the hands in Anjali Mudra (prayer position). This can be a balancing posture on its own. Breathe freely.

Position 2: If you are feeling more adventurous, then inhale, and exhale as you start to tilt forward and straighten the left leg, stretching the arms behind the body as if you are flying, keeping the gaze forward. Hold for a few seconds. Breathe freely.

Position 3: Then inhale and slowly bring the arms forward, placing the palms in Anjali Mudra once more, and exhale as you drop into the half squat.

Repeat to the other side.

Benefits: Helps balance the nervous system, and strengthens the legs, hips and spine. Improves balance and concentration.

Cautions: Can be a problem for weak ankles.

As we age, being able to balance is extremely important. Many difficulties can arise if we lose this abililty.

Although balances can be quite difficult to perform, especially if we come to them later in life, great progress can be made after a few weeks of practice.

The focus we develop in performing these asanas not only balances the physical body, but also give us balance at a mental and emotional level.

Vajrasana – *Thunderbolt Pose*

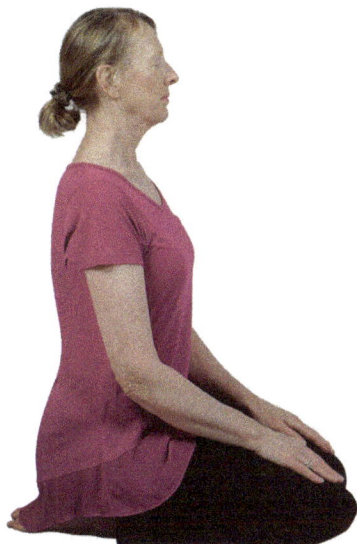

This posture is the starting position for many of the kneeling poses.

From kneeling, bring the big toes together and separate the heels. Lower the buttocks on to the inside surface of the feet with the heels touching the sides of the hips. Place the hands on the knees, palms facing down.

Lift and lengthen the spine. The back and head should be in alignment. Avoid excessive backward arching of the spine.

Close the eyes, relax the arms and the whole body. Breathe normally and keep the awareness on the breath.

Benefits: Vajrasana is a meditation posture as it helps the body to remain upright and straight, allowing space for the lungs to expand and for the body to breathe freely.

As this pose stretches the vajra nadi (thunderbolt channel), it also increases the efficiency of the entire digestive system.

Cautions: Not appropriate for people with knee problems or varicose veins.

Pranatasana – *Pose of the Child*

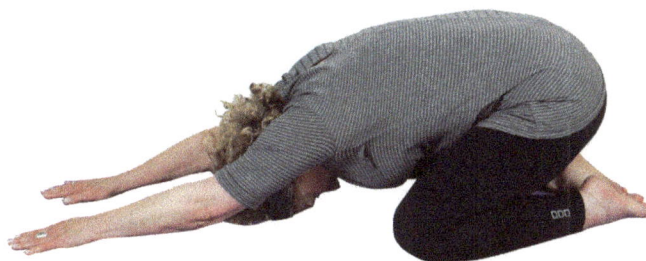

This is a commonly used counterpose, especially after back bending asanas, when your body can surrender to gravity and say 'yes' to letting go.

Sit in Vajrasana. Exhale, fold from the hips to place the forehead on the floor, arms back alongside the body, palms facing upwards or downwards to release the fingers and wrists.

Breathe freely and feel yourself internalising, and the body relaxing.

Tip: After strong poses, stretch the arms out on the floor in front and walk the fingers away from the body to stretch through the spine. Focus on the breath.

Modifications: ❁ If you have high blood pressure, make two fists with the hands, place them one on top of the other and rest your forehead on the uppermost fist.

Also use this modification if your buttocks do not rest on your heels.

If the pressure is too much on your abdomen when you fold forward, then sit with the knees hip-width apart.

Benefits: Calms the mind. Neutralises the spine after back bending. Releases shoulders.

Simhasana – *Lion Pose*

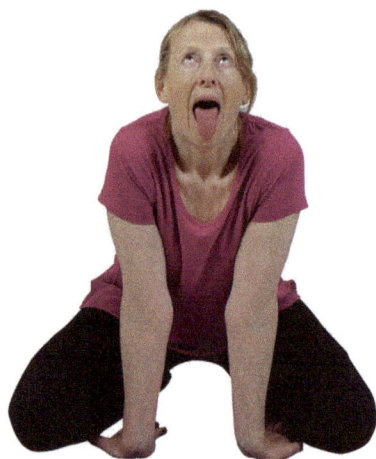

Begin in Vajrasana.

Place the palms of the hands on the floor between the knees, with the fingers pointing towards the body Keep the arms straight. Tilt forward, resting the body weight on the hands.

Eyes open, gaze at the eyebrow centre or the tip of the nose. Relax the body.

Inhale slowly and deeply through the nose. At the completion of the inhalation, open the mouth and extend the tongue as far as possible to the chin. While slowly exhaling, make a steady, constant, loud '*aaaahh*' sound from the throat.

When inhalation is necessary, retract the tongue, close the lips and eyes, and feel the release of tension throughout the whole body.

This is round one. Complete several rounds.

Modification: ❀ Place hands on the knees instead of on the floor.

Benefits: May relieve conditions of the throat, nose, ears, eyes and mouth. Removes tension from the chest and diaphragm. Works the abdominal organs.

Anjaneyasana – *Lunge Pose*

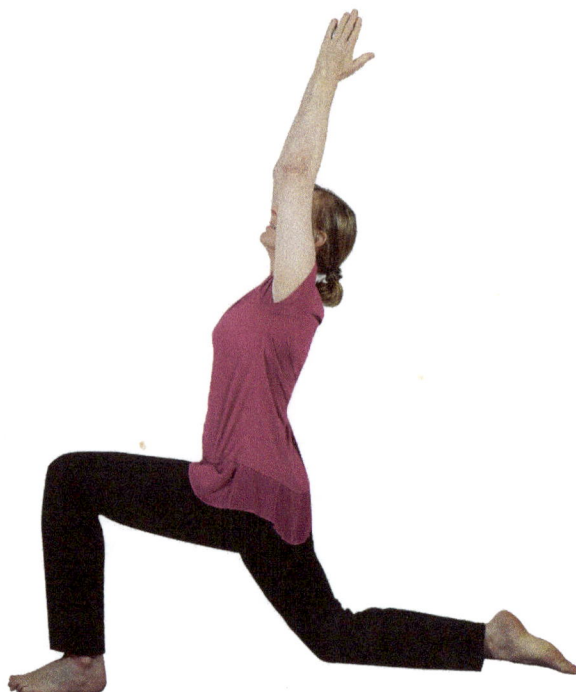

Begin from a kneeling position.

Inhale and step the right foot forward. The right leg should be straight. Place the hands loosely on the right thigh, or on the hips.

Exhale and lunge, so that the right leg is at a right angle, the knee over the ankle. At the same time raise the arms over the head, vertical and parallel with palms facing. Lift up out of the pelvis, lengthening the spine.

The hips remain facing forward. Look straight ahead or tilt the head a little to look up at the hands. Breathe freely.

To release, inhale and straighten the leg, then exhale bringing the arms back down beside the body and return to kneeling.

Repeat to the other side.

Counterpose: ⟳

Benefits: Strengthens legs, spine, shoulders. Brings flexibility to the hips. Expands the chest and lungs bringing life force into the body.

In order to see, you have to stop being in the middle of the picture.

– Sri Aurobindo

Ardha Ustrasana – *Half Camel Pose*

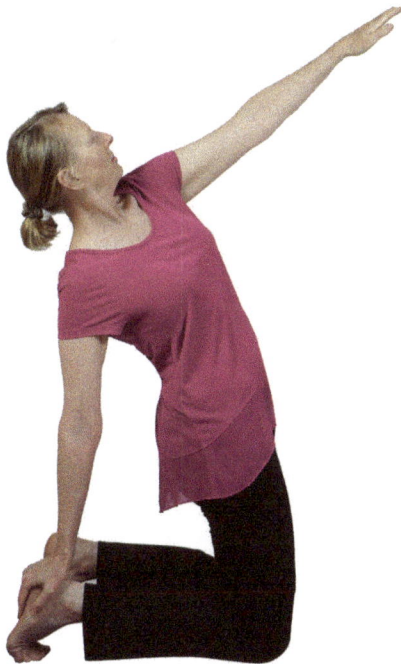

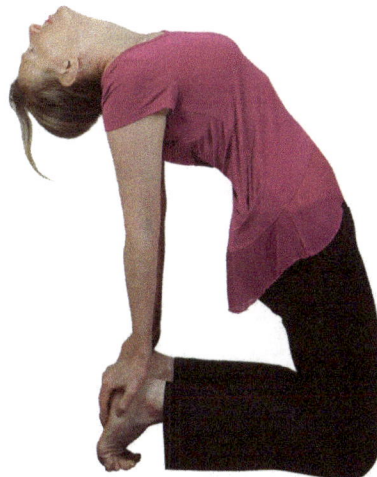

Commence from a kneeling position.

Have the knees hip-width apart. The feet can be flat to the floor, or turn the toes under and lift the heels off the floor.

Inhale, float the arms up to shoulder height and lengthen through the spine.

Exhale, turn to look behind you and place the right hand on the right heel, then look to the front and bring the left arm to eyebrow level.

Gently push the thighs forward to vertical. Inhale, raise the left arm. The head should be slightly back with the eyes gazing at the raised left arm. Breathe freely.

Repeat to the other side.

Modification: ✺ Place hands on the hips, lengthening through the body. Tilt slightly backwards and gently push the thighs forward to vertical.

Counterpose:

Benefits: Beneficial for the digestive system. Stretches the vertebrae stimulating the spinal nerves. Works the adrenals and expands the chest.

Cautions: Not appropriate if there are any back or neck problems, or enlarged thyroid.

Ustrasana – *Camel Pose*

Commence from a kneeling position.

Knees are hip-width apart. The feet can be flat to the floor, or turn the toes under and lift the heels off the floor.

Inhale, float the arms up to shoulder height and lengthen through the spine. Exhale, turn to look behind and place the right hand on the right foot, then look back to the front and bring the left hand to the left foot.

Gently push the thighs forward to vertical. The head should gently tilt backwards. The weight of the body should be evenly supported by the arms and legs.

Modification: ✺ As per Ardha Ustrasana (left).

Counterpose:

Benefits: Beneficial for the digestive system. It stretches the vertebrae stimulating the spinal nerves. Works the adrenals and expands the chest. The front of the neck being fully stretched helps to regulate the thyroid gland.

Cautions: Not appropriate if there are any back or neck problems, or enlarged thyroid.

Parighasana – *Gate Pose*

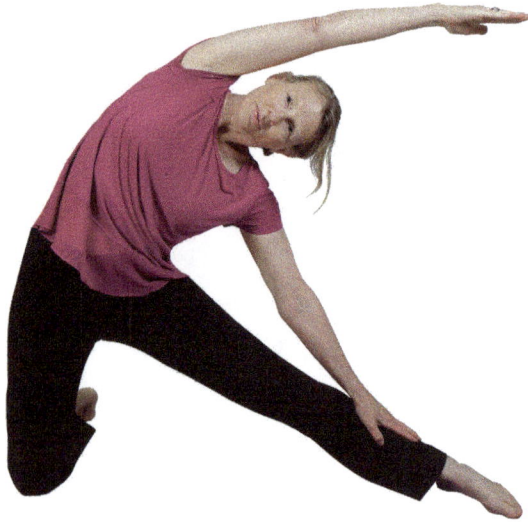

Counterpose for Parighasana

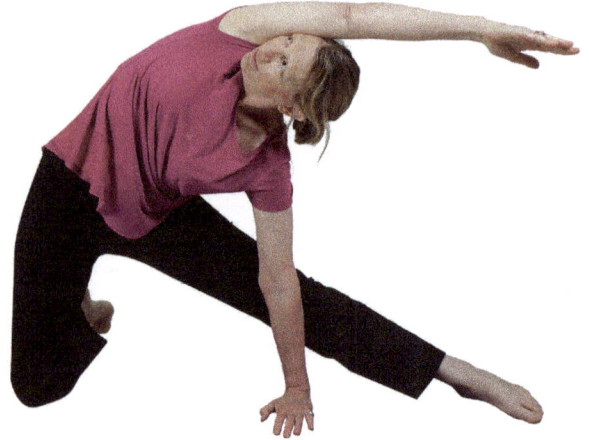

Begin kneeling.

Inhale, stretch the right leg sideways to the right, in line with the hips, right foot flat to the floor turning the toes in slightly. Keep the hips facing forward.

Exhale, then inhale and raise the left arm towards the ceiling. Place right palm on the right thigh. Exhale, extend the body to the right, the right palm sliding down the right leg to rest at the ankle the left arm resting close to the left ear. Look ahead or turn the head to look up to the raised left arm. Try not to roll the left shoulder forward – keep it in line with the right arm and right leg.

Breathe freely.

To release out of the pose, inhale, raise the arms out to the sides at shoulder height, then exhale and lower the arms.

Counterpose: This beautiful lateral stretch has its own counterpose in the next column.

Modification: ✺ Bring the right palm to the shin or knee, left arm to vertical.

Benefits: Strong lateral stretch for the spine, opens the chest, strengthens the abdomen, hips and legs.

Cautions: Be careful with knee and lower back problems.

Parighasana has an inbuilt counterpose.

After performing the lateral stretch to the left, inhale and stretch the right arm overhead alongside the ear, then exhale and place the left hand on the floor, level with the left knee, fingers facing forward.

Stretch through the whole right side of the body by pushing the right foot to the floor, and keeping the right arm engaged, fingers stretched. The body is in a straight line from the right foot through the trunk of the body and out to the fingertips.

Breathe freely.

Parighasana and the counterpose form half a round. Change the position of the legs and repeat to the other side.

Modification: ✺ If you can't reach to place the left hand on the floor, then place the arm alongside the left thigh, and lean to the left as you raise the right arm overhead and alongside the right ear.

Benefits: Strong lateral stretch for the spine, opens the chest, strengthens the abdomen, hips and legs.

Cautions: Be careful with knee and lower back problems.

Sasamgasana – *Hare Pose*

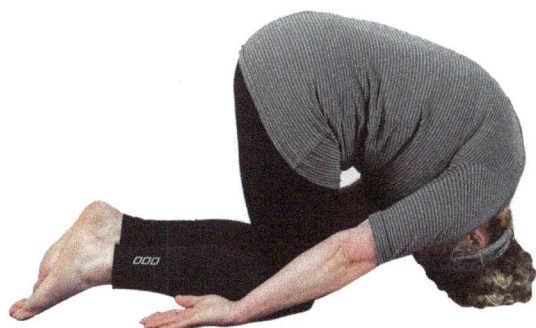

Sit in Vajrasana.

Take hold the heels with the thumbs to the outside of feet. Exhale, bring the chin to the chest and continue to curl forward until the top of your head touches the floor, preferably on a folded blanket.

Then begin to lift your hips up from the heels until the thighs are as close to vertical as is comfortable. Gently walk your knees a little closer to the forehead, making sure to go only as far as feels comfortable. Place the minimum amount of weight on the head and neck.

Breathe freely – hold the pose for about 20 seconds, and on an inhalation, firstly return to the extended pose of the child for a short time, and then return to Vajrasana.

Modification: ✿ Place hands a little forward of either side of the knees before bringing the head to the floor.

Counterpose:

Benefits: Increases the blood supply to the head and neck. Decompresses the neck vertebrae, releasing tension in the neck and spine. The upper back and shoulders are stretched.

Caution: Avoid this asana if you have untreated blood pressure, ear and eye disorders or neck problems.

Threading the Needle

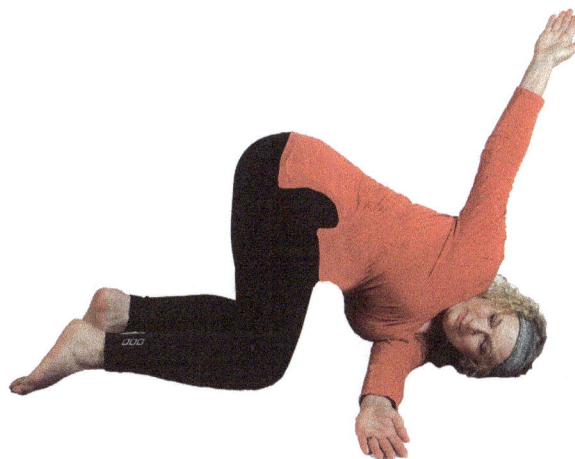

Start this posture on hands and knees, hands placed straight below the shoulders and the knees beneath the hips.

Inhale, and as you exhale, bring your left shoulder to the floor and stretch your arm in front of your body with the palm facing upwards. Stretch your left arm out to the side so that you can place the right and left palms together.

Make sure you are stable. Inhale and raise the right arm to vertical – follow the hand with your eyes. Stretch the right arm back strongly so you can feel the expansion in the chest.

You can do this pose statically (holding the pose) or dynamically (doing several at a time with the breath).

Repeat to the other side.

Modification: This is a strong stretch for the shoulder and you may have to work on your flexibility in this area before you can manage this pose.

Counterpose:

Benefits: This pose relieves tension in the upper body, especially the chest and between the shoulder blades. It gives a great lateral stretch for the rib cage and a soft, spinal twist.

Cautions: Avoid if you have any neck or shoulder problems.

Vyaghrasana – *Tiger Pose*

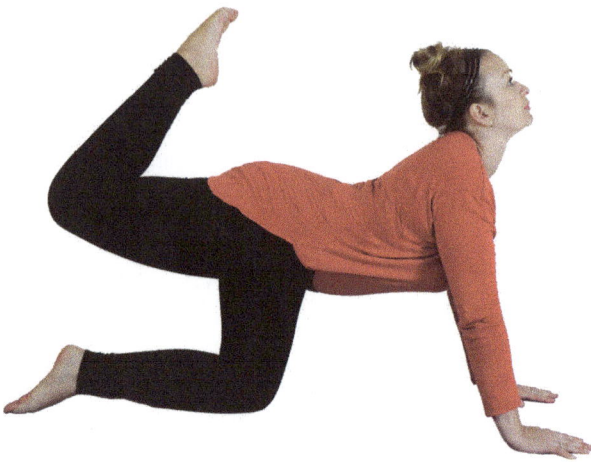

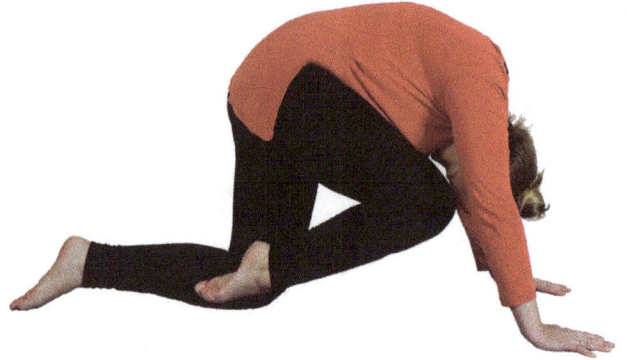

Start this posture on hands and knees.

Hands are underneath the shoulders, the arms and thighs perpendicular to the floor. The hands should be in line with the knees. The arms are shoulder-width apart and the knees are a little less than hip-width apart.

Relax the whole body. Inhale, lift the head and straighten the right leg back behind. Bend the right knee and form a right angle with the leg. Hold the breath here for a few seconds.

Exhale and straighten the right leg, arch the back, bend the knee and swing the leg under the hips and lower the head to the knee. The right foot should not touch the floor.

The knee should press against the chest and the spine should be rounded into a convex shape. Hold the breath here for a few seconds.

Continue with this movement 6 times to each side.

Modification: ✹ The benefits of this asana come from the movement of the spine from one extreme to the other and it is not important if your head and knee do not meet.

Counterpose: There is no need to counterpose this asana but it feels nice to drop back into Extended Pose of the Child.

Benefits: This asana tones the spinal nerves as it gently undulates the spine from one direction to another. It helps to relieve sciatica and it relaxes the legs. It is also good for the digestive system and stimulates blood circulation.

Through the practice of yoga, the tensions are removed and the stage dawns where there is an end to this eternal struggle within.

This is the stage of sublime equanimity.

– Swami Satyananda Saraswati

Chatuspadasana – *Quadruped Pose*

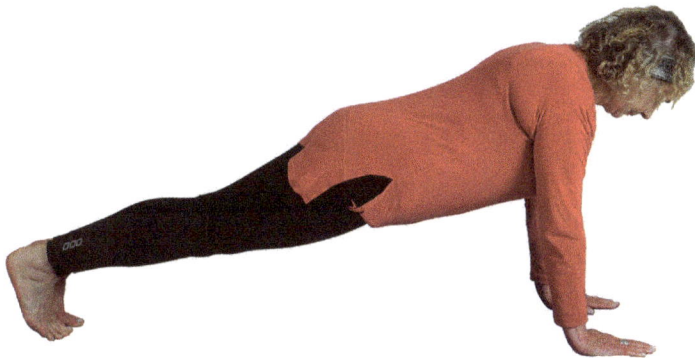

Chest Opening Lateral Stretch

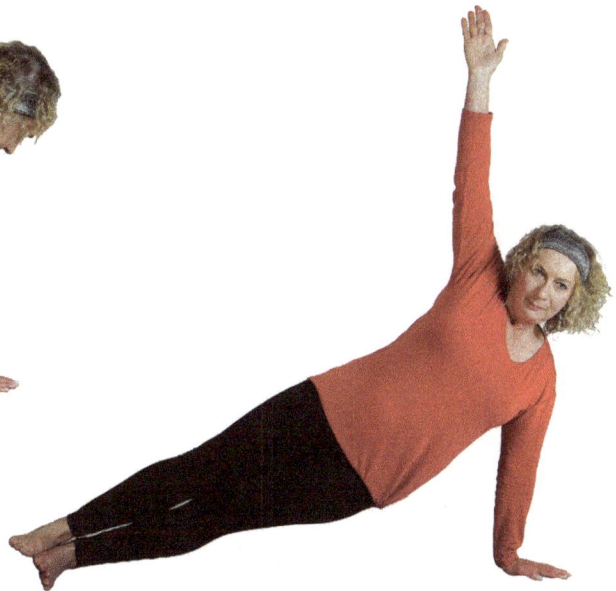

Start this posture on hands and knees, hands placed underneath the shoulders and knees beneath the hips.

Inhale, slide the right leg straight back behind and exhale. Inhale, slide the left leg straight back behind. Tuck toes under. Make sure the arms are vertical to the floor, wrists under the shoulders, fingers pointing forward. The head, neck and spine are in a straight line.

Make the abdomen firm and breathe freely.

Maintain a straight line with the body, making sure the buttocks are not raised and that the abdomen is not sinking towards the floor.

Hold as long as is comfortable.

To release, exhale and bring the knees to the floor.

Slide back into Extended Pose of the Child.

Benefits: Strengthens the whole body and is good for weight-bearing in the upper body.

Cautions: Can be a problem for weak wrists. Care should also be taken if there are shoulder problems.

Start this posture on hands and knees, hands placed straight below the shoulders and the knees beneath the hips.

Move the right hand and right knee to the centre of the body and turn the bottom half of the right leg out to the side. This acts as a rudder.

Inhale, and slowly raise the left arm to vertical, opening out to the side. The arms form one vertical line. Feel the chest opening, and the lateral stretch down the left side of the body. Feel the stretch invite the rib cage to softly open.

Exhale return to the starting position and repeat 6 times.

Then repeat 6 times to the other side.

Counterpose:

Benefits: This pose relieves tension in the upper body, particularly the chest and the shoulder blades. It opens the sides of the rib cage and is also a gentle spinal twist.

Cautions: Care should be taken if you have shoulder problems or weak wrists.

Marjariasana – *Cat Pose*

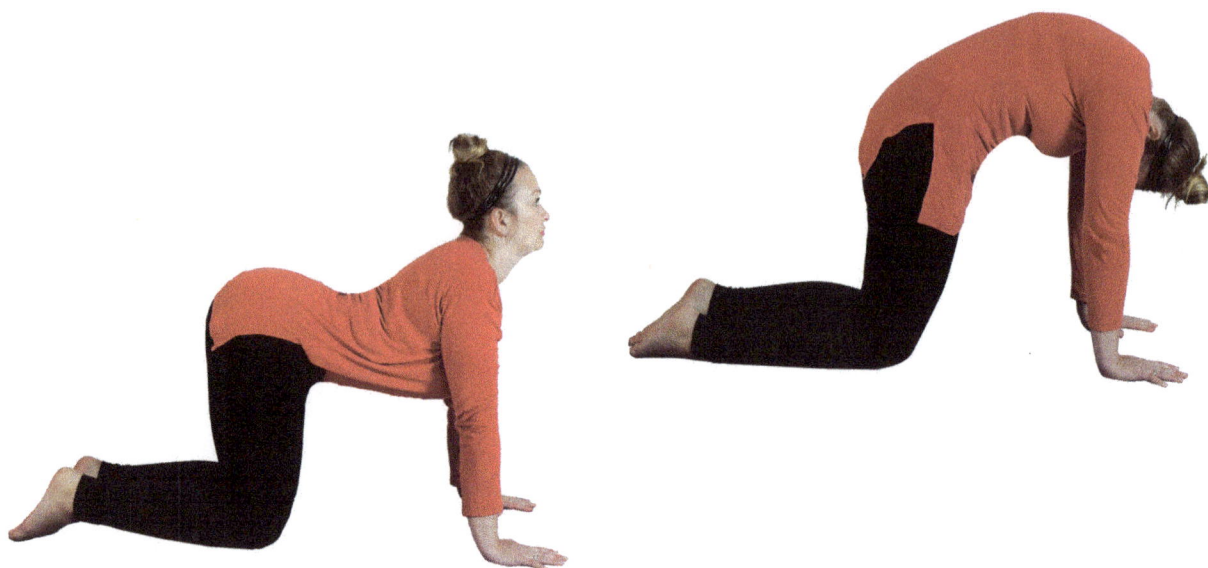

Start this posture on hands and knees.

Hands are underneath the shoulders. The arms and thighs are perpendicular to the floor. The hands should be in line with the knees. The arms are shoulder-width apart and the knees are hip-width apart. Spread the fingers to distribute the body weight evenly. Have the inner elbows facing each other.

Inhale and raise the head and depress the spine so that the back becomes concave. Fill the lungs with the maximum amount of air. Hold the breath for approximately the count of 3.

Exhale, bring the chin towards the chest, draw the abdomen towards the spine, tuck the tail-bone under, squeeze the buttocks together, and hunch up like a cat arching. The head will now be between the arms, facing the thighs. Hold the breath out for approximately the count of 3. (One can also do some pelvic floor exercise on the exhalation by drawing the perineum upwards into the body, and releasing on the inhalation).

Gently undulate the spine as you move through inhalation to exhalation, making a smooth, wavelike movement with the spine.

Benefits: This asana is especially beneficial as it can be done by anyone. Its gentle, relaxed rhythm belies its effectiveness, especially in keeping the spine supple.

This asana is the standout asana in any yoga class. It doesn't foster competitiveness in any way – not even with yourself.

You will note there are no contraindications. The pose is so gentle there is no need to counterpose, although sliding back on the heels afterwards and having a long stretch of the spine in Extended Pose of the Child seems to complete the pose.

As human beings, our greatness lies not so much in being able to remake the world ... as in being able to remake ourselves.

– Mahatma Gandhi

Gomukhasana – *Face of a Cow Pose*

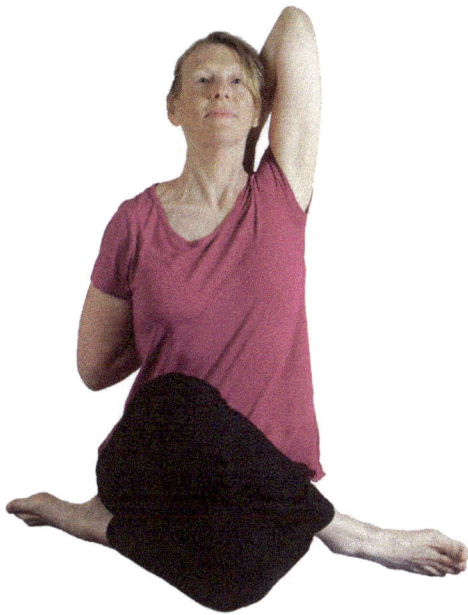

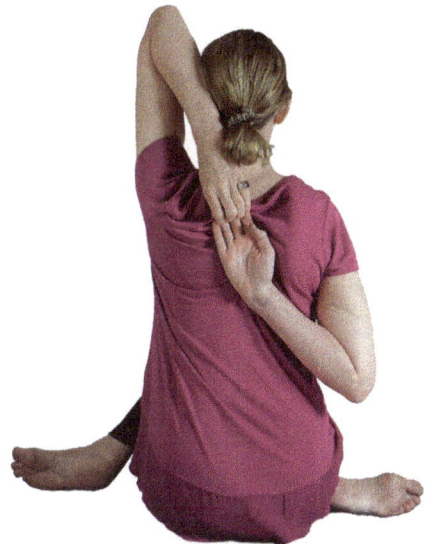

Rear view

Sit in Dandasana (see the following page) and come into a kneeling position. Then drape the right leg in front of the left and lower back to a seated position, with the knees stacked one on top of the other. The feet are at right angles to the body and evenly placed on either side.

Inhale, raise the left arm out to the side, the thumb pointing towards the floor. Exhale, slide that arm up the back of the body between the shoulder blades as high as you can manage. Inhale and lengthen the right arm over the head, bend the elbow to hook the fingers of the hands together. Keep the spine straight or lean back slightly, chin tucked in, and the right arm alongside the ear. Focus on the breath and breathe freely.

To come out of the pose, exhale and release the arms and legs. Repeat to the other side.

Modifications: ❀ To modify the leg position you can fold the right leg under the body and have the heel in the perineum, then drape the left leg over the right thigh. Another modification with the legs is to sit in Vajrasana or kneel on the floor. If your fingers don't reach, then use a belt or sock.

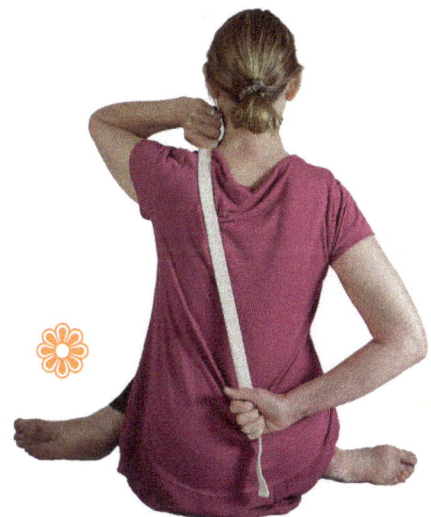

Using a belt

Benefits: This pose can help with sciatica but only if you can move into the leg position without stressing the body. Go gently. This pose works the shoulders, arms, and opens the chest area to help improve breathing. It also works the spine, hips and legs.

Cautions: Not appropriate if you have trouble with shoulders, hips or knees and ankles. Modify.

Dandasana – *Rod Pose*

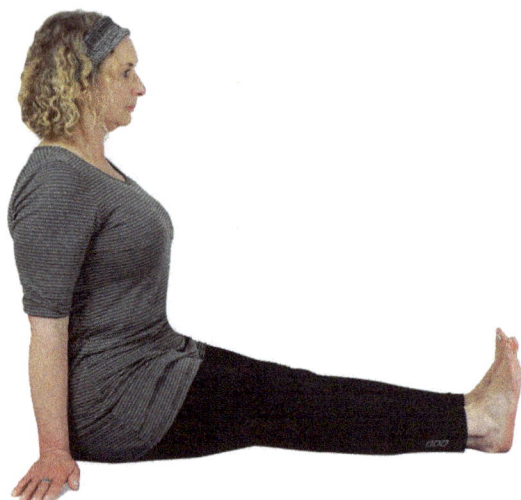

Purvottanasana – *Backward Plank Pose*

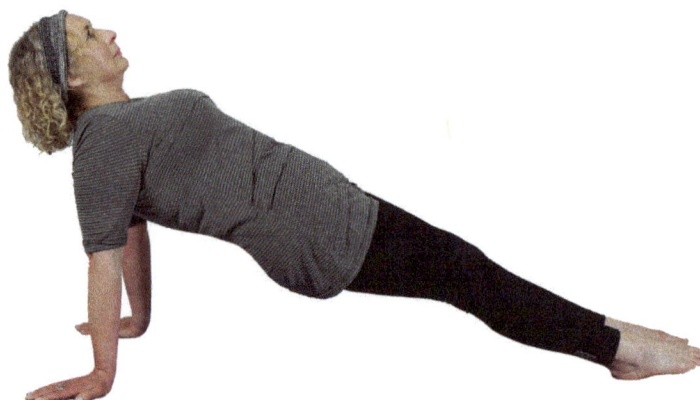

Many of the seated poses start in Dandasana.

It is important to sit on the thighs and sitting bones in this posture – not on the coccyx (tailbone). To do this, push the hands against the floor to lift the hips off the floor and move them back behind you, tilting the body forward slightly. Gently lower back down to the floor.

Have the knees and ankles together and stretch the backs of the legs on the floor, extending the hamstrings. Flex the feet towards the face. The chin is parallel to the floor.

Draw the kneecaps back towards the groin, engaging the quadricep muscles. The hands are beside the hips with the fingers facing outwards. Push down through the hands to lengthen through the spine. Roll the shoulders back and down.

Hold for 10 breaths or more.

Benefits: Stretches the hamstring muscles in preparation for forward bending asana, and strengthens the back, abdomen, legs and feet.

In Dandasana the body is in perfect, seated alignment.

Start in Dandasana.

Lean back and place the hands behind the body underneath the shoulders, the fingers pointing forwards. On an inhalation, stretch the legs, firm the abdomen and lengthen through the body. Raise the pelvis and chest off the floor.

Bring the souls of the feet to the floor.

Do not allow the head to drop too far backwards; keep it in line with the spine.

In the mind's eye, picture the body in a straight line from the head to the toes.

Breathe freely.

Hold while comfortable and on an exhalation, lower the body to the floor.

Benefits: Strengthens the abdominal muscles, shoulders, arms, wrists and back. Great weight bearing for the upper body.

Cautions: Can be difficult if you have weak wrists.

Paschimottanasana – *Forward Stretch Pose*

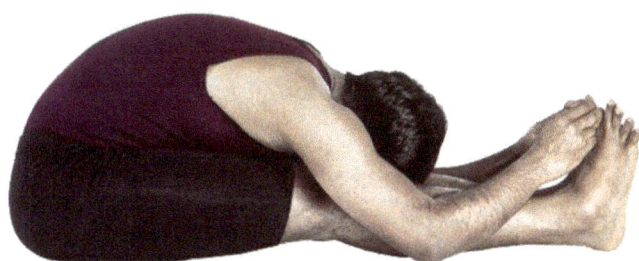

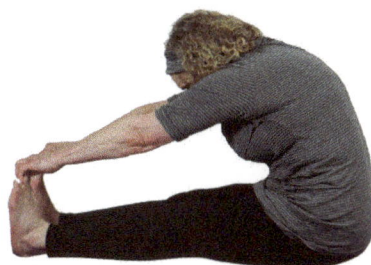
Fig. 1

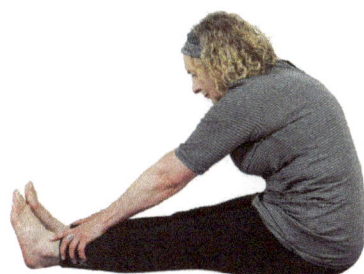
Fig. 2

It is important to sit on the thighs and sitting bones in this posture – not on the coccyx (tailbone). To do this, sit in Dandasana and push the hands against the floor to lift the hips off the floor and move them back behind you, tilting the body forward slightly. Gently lower back down to the floor.

Inhale, raise the arms over the head, lift up tall to lengthen through the spine. Exhale, draw in the abdominal muscles, fold forward from the hips (not the waist) and take hold of the big toes with the fingers, or the heels or ankles. Tuck the chin in slightly. Bring the head down towards the knees, touching if possible.

To release, roll to upright, sliding the hands along the legs. Inhale and raise the arms overhead, exhale and release the arms back to the sides of the body.

Modifications: ✱ Sit on the edge of a folded blanket to aid tilting forward and to support the back. If you can't bring the head down to knees then tilt forward to your limit, but do not strain (Fig. 1). If you cannot reach the toes, then reach the ankles (Fig. 2). Place a belt around the feet and slowly inch your fingers down the belt until you are tilted forward (Fig. 3). For full support, bend knees and bring thighs to the chest, hands around the shins. Slowly slide feet forward on the floor and stop when the chest starts to leave the thighs.

Counterpose: ⟢ or 🧍

Benefits: Stretches the hamstring muscles and increases flexibility in the hip joints and spine. It also massages the abdominal and pelvic areas.

Cautions: Do not bounce the body back and forth trying to reach the toes. This is extremely harmful to the spine. If you have disc problems then this pose is not for you. If you have issues with sciatica, then modify by bending knees.

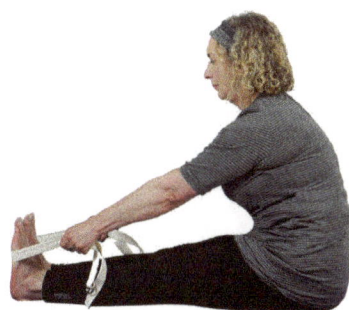
Fig. 3

Nothing would be done at all if a man waited until he could do it so well that no-one could find fault with it.

– Cardinal Newman

37

Janu Sirshasana – *Head to Knee Pose*

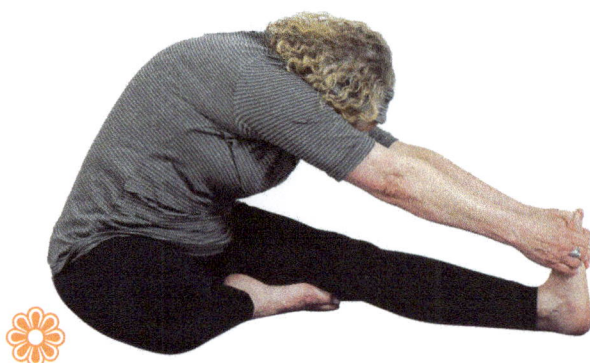

Easy Seated Spinal Twist

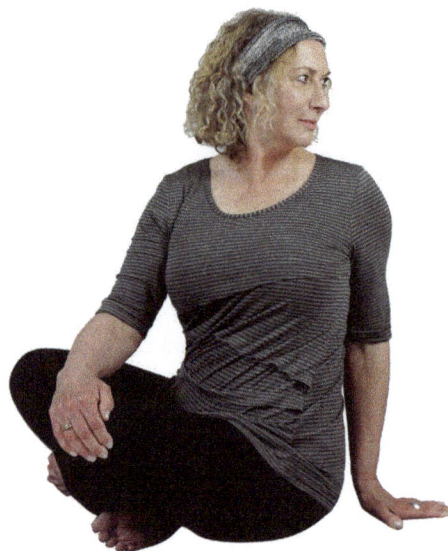

Start in Dandasana and ensure you are not sitting on your tail bone.

Bend the left leg and place the sole of the foot against the inside of the right thigh, knee to the floor.

Inhale, raise the arms overhead, palms facing, and lengthen through the spine. Exhale, engage the abdominal muscles, fold forward from the hips and bring the hands towards the extended foot. Inhale, lift and lengthen further through the body, and exhale, lower the body to the thigh.

Hold for as long as is comfortable. Inhaling, slide the hands up the inside of the extended leg, then raise them out to the sides at shoulder height, and on an exhalation lower the arms.

Modification: ❋ Bring hands to the feet but do not lower body to thigh (as shown in above image).

Counterpose:

Benefits: Stretches the hamstring muscles and increases flexibility in the hip joints and spine. It also massages the abdominal and pelvic areas. Not for SI joint problems.*

Cautions: Do not practice this pose if you have disc or sciatica problems.

*Sacroiliac Joint Dysfunction

Sit in an easy pose (legs crossed loosely at the ankles).

Place right hand on left knee, and left hand at the base of spine.

Inhale, stretch up tall, exhale, twist the head and upper trunk to look over the left shoulder. Hold, then inhale and return to centre.

Relax and breathe freely in this position. Eyes are closed and the focus is on the breath.

Hold for approximately the count of 10 and repeat to the other side.

Counterpose: Stretch the arms out in front of the body, fingertips on the floor and stretch forward.

Benefits: Gentle twist for the body.

Cautions: Go gently if you have lower back problems.

Regrets are baggage that will only slow you down. You cannot go back to rectify your mistakes. Learn from them, and then leave them where they fell. The road runs ahead of you, not behind you.

– Wilbur Smith

Matsyendrasana – *Lord of the Fish Pose*

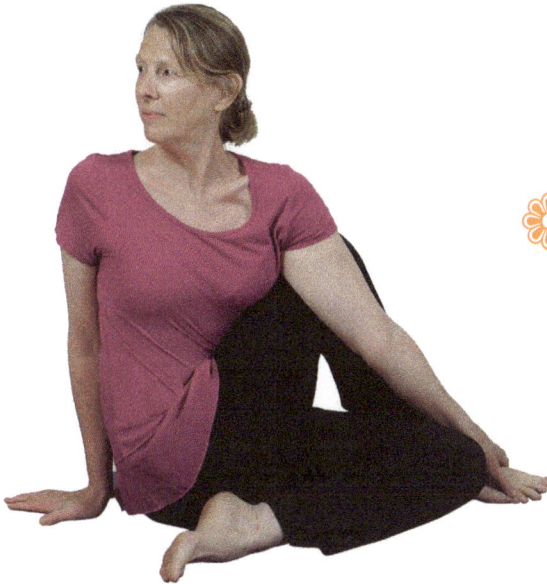

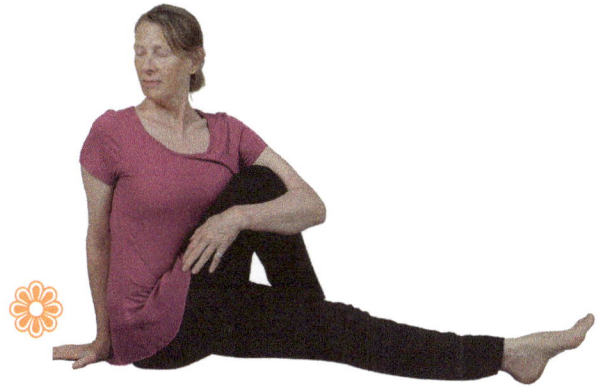

Sit in Dandasana. Draw the left knee towards the chest, and step the left leg over the right leg in line with the knee. Fold the right leg and sweep leg behind the body with the heel in line with the left buttocks.

Relax and inhale. Exhale and place the right upper arm on the outer side of the left thigh and hold the left foot.

Inhale, lengthen the spine and make sure the pelvis is facing forward and both buttocks are on the floor.

Place the left hand behind the body at the base of the spine, palm flat to the floor. Inhale and slowly turn the trunk to look over the left shoulder and then turn the head. Keep shoulders level and ears away from the shoulders.

Hold for as long as is comfortable, breathing freely.

To release, inhale, and on the exhalation, return the head to the front and then release the trunk and arms and legs. Repeat to the other side.

Modifications: ❀ If both buttocks are not on the floor, then keep one leg straight out in front. If the folded arm cannot reach the foot, then have the arm at a right angle, palm facing forward.

If you cannot get the arm on the outer side of the opposite thigh, then fold the arm around the lifted leg.

Counterpose: This or

Benefits: Massages abdominal organs, stimulates spine, adrenal glands, kidneys, pancreas.

Cautions: Care should be taken with lower back problem or osteoporosis.

If you practise yoga every day with perseverance, you will be able to face the turmoil of life with steadiness and maturity.

– BKS Iyengar

❀

In reality spirituality is not about glamour, intensity or escapist meditation but about being fully present in every moment to moment relationship and situation.

– Bernard Gunther

Shavasana – *Corpse Pose*

Advasana – *Prone Corpse Pose*

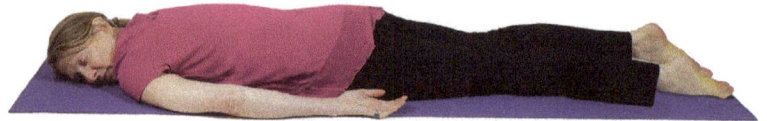

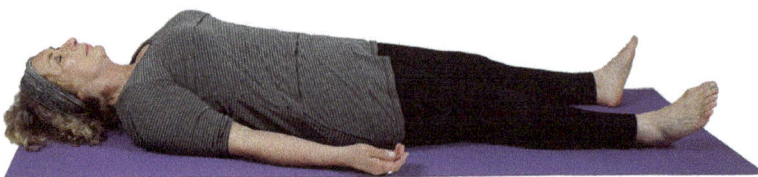

Lie on the floor with the feet hip-width apart, feet flopping to the outside. Have the arms alongside the body, but not touching the body.

The head and neck are in a straight line with the spine. The palms of the hands face upwards, the fingers lightly curled. The palms roll a little inwards towards the body.

Tuck the chin in slightly to avoid an uncomfortable arch in the neck.

Focus on relaxing the body. On each out breath, feel the body releasing, relaxing, melting down and letting go.

Modification: ✿ If you experience pain in the lower back after lying for any length of time, place a rolled blanket or cushion under the thighs or knees.

Benefits: Total body and mind relaxation. This asana can be used as a counterpose for any strong asana.

The art of lying in Shavasana is described in full on page 75.

Advasana is the resting position for many of the back bending asanas that commence from the prone position.

Lie on the front of the body, head turned to one side. Arms are alongside the body but not touching the body, with the palms facing upwards. Relax the elbows. The heels drop outwards.

Lie for equal amounts of time with the head on either side.

Benefits: Relaxation of the body/mind.

Can be used between strong asana practices to relax and bring the body back to a neutral position.

Within you there is a stillness and a sanctuary to which you can retreat at any time and be yourself.

– Herman Hesse (Siddhartha)

Dhanurasana – *Bow Pose*

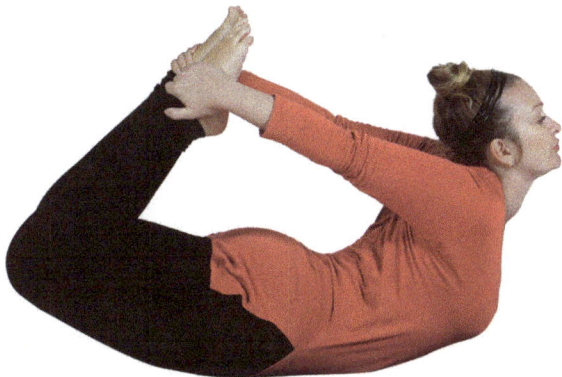

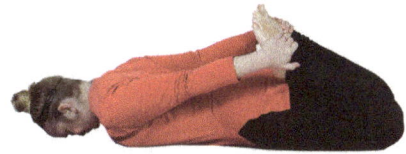

Fig. 1

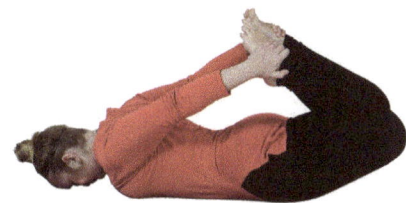

Fig. 2

Start in Advasana. Place the forehead on the floor.

Bend the knees and bring the heels close to the buttocks. Reach behind and place the hands around the outside of the ankles.

Inhale and push the feet back into the hands and lift legs up and away from the floor to raise the thighs, head and chest off the floor. Tuck the chin in slightly and draw the shoulders back. The body is balanced on the abdomen. It is important to keep the knees and ankles in line with the hips.

Modification 1: For some people, just reaching around to take hold of the ankles is a sufficient stretch in this pose until the body is strong and flexible enough to do the full pose (Fig. 1).

Modification 2: If Modification 1 is do-able without causing knee problems, then push the feet back into the hands and draw the legs away from the body to raise the thighs from the floor, but allow the head and chest to stay on the floor (Fig.2).

Counterpose: This then

Benefits: The spine, shoulders, hips and thighs become stronger and more flexible.

Cautions: Avoid this pose altogether if there are knee problems. Care should be taken if there are back problems.

Happiness is a butterfly which, when pursued, is always just beyond your grasp but which, if you sit down quietly, may light upon you.

– Nathaniel Hawthorne

Sarpasana – *Snake Pose*

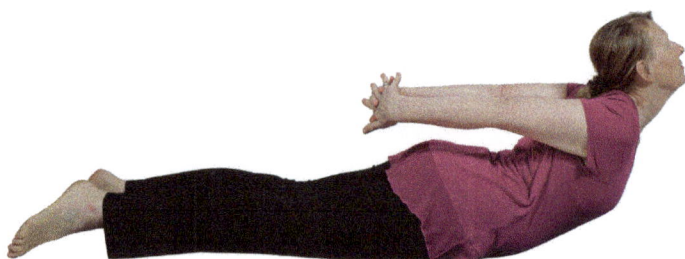

Sphinx

Start in Advasana. Place the chin on the floor. Feet are together. Interlock the hands on top of the body.

Inhale, using the lower back muscles, raise the head and chest off the floor and raise the arms up and back behind as far as possible. Raise the body as high as possible but do not force. Squeeze the shoulder blades together.

Look straight ahead, chin slightly tucked in.

Hold the breath for the duration of the pose and then on an exhalation, lower the body back to Advasana. Relax the whole body and release the hands. Turn the head to one side. Repeat once more, and on completion, turn the head to the opposite side.

Counterpose: This ⌒ then ⌒

Benefits: Works the shoulder, arms, back, spine, legs. It opens the chest and the breath retention works the lungs.

Cautions: Not to be practised if there is a heart condition or high blood pressure.

Note: In some traditions, the legs are also raised off the floor, with the body balanced on the abdomen.

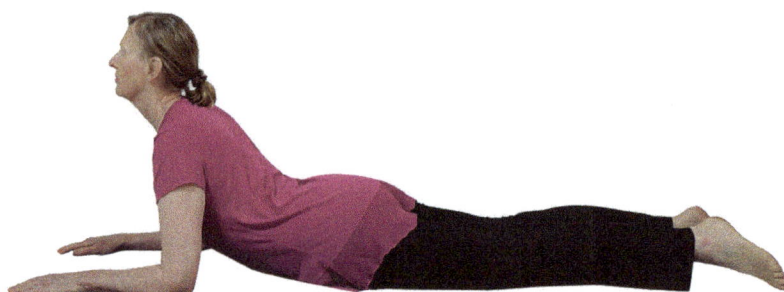

Start in Advasana. Place the forehead on the floor. Feet are hip-width apart, soles of the feet uppermost.

Bend the elbows and place the forearms on the floor with the palms facing downward. The forearms and elbows are held close to the body. The fingertips point forward but are in line with the crown of the head.

Inhale, raise the chest and head by bringing the upper arms to vertical, the elbows and forearms remain on the floor. The elbows are below the shoulders, the arms forming a right angle.

Roll the shoulders down the back, ensuring the ears are well away from the shoulders. Tuck the chin in a little to avoid creating an uncomfortable arch in the neck. The chest is open and the eyes look straight ahead.

Breathe freely.

Stay in this position for a comfortable length of time, and then slowly lower back down to Advasana.

Counterpose: This ⌒ then ⌒

Benefits: Brings flexibility to the back and spine. Opens the chest. Beneficial for the kidneys and adrenal glands.

Bhujangasana – *Cobra Pose*

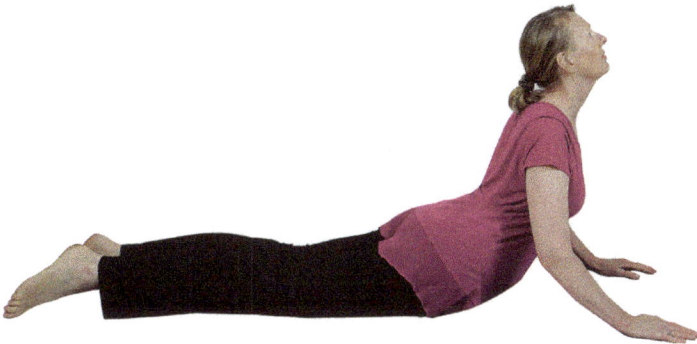

Urdhva Mukha Savasana –
Upward Facing Dog Pose

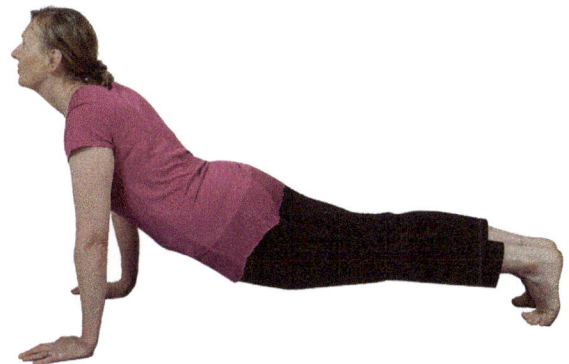

Start in Advasana. Place the forehead on the floor. Feet are hip-width apart, soles of the feet uppermost.

Bend the elbows and place the palms of the hands on the floor under the shoulders. The elbows point backwards and hug the body. Rest the forehead on the floor and relax the whole body, especially the lower back.

Inhale, slowly start to lift the forehead, then nose, then chin and shoulders off the floor, followed by the chest. The navel is off the floor, but the pubic bone is still on the floor. Use the back muscles to lift off the floor and when they can't take you further, use the arm muscles.

Focus straight ahead with the chin tucked in slightly. For some people the arms will be straight, for others the elbows will be bent. Hold for the duration of the inhalation, then exhale and lower back down to Advasana.

Modifications: ✺ For lower back problems, only go as far as the Sphinx Pose (see previous page).

Counterpose: This ◁▱ then ◁৲

Benefits: Works the back, spine and opens the chest. Beneficial for kidneys and adrenals.

Cautions: Not appropriate for some back conditions but can be beneficial for others. You need to monitor how you feel after completing this pose and act accordingly.

Start in Advasana. Place the forehead on the floor. Feet are hip-width apart, soles of the feet uppermost or toes curled under.

Bend the elbows and place the palms of the hands on the floor, the wrists level with the ribs. The elbows point backwards and hug the body. Bring the forehead to floor.

Inhale, slowly start to lift the head, chest, shoulders and trunk off the floor until the arms are straight. Press the toes or tops of the feet firmly into the floor to lift the shins, knees, thighs and pubic bone off the floor. Exhale, press down into the hands to lift the body and push forward with the chest. Keep the shoulders relaxed, ears well away from the shoulders. Maintain the forward and upward lift of the chest. Hold for as long as is comfortable, breathing freely.

Exhale and lower to the floor in Advasana.

Modifications: ✺ For lower back problems, only go as far as the Sphinx Pose (see previous page).

Counterpose: This ◁▱ then ◁৲

Benefits: Works the back, spine and opens the chest. Beneficial for kidneys and adrenals.

Cautions: Do not practise this pose if you have lower back problems, shoulder or wrist problems.

Adha Salabhasana – *Half Locust Pose*   ## Salabhasana – *Locust Pose*

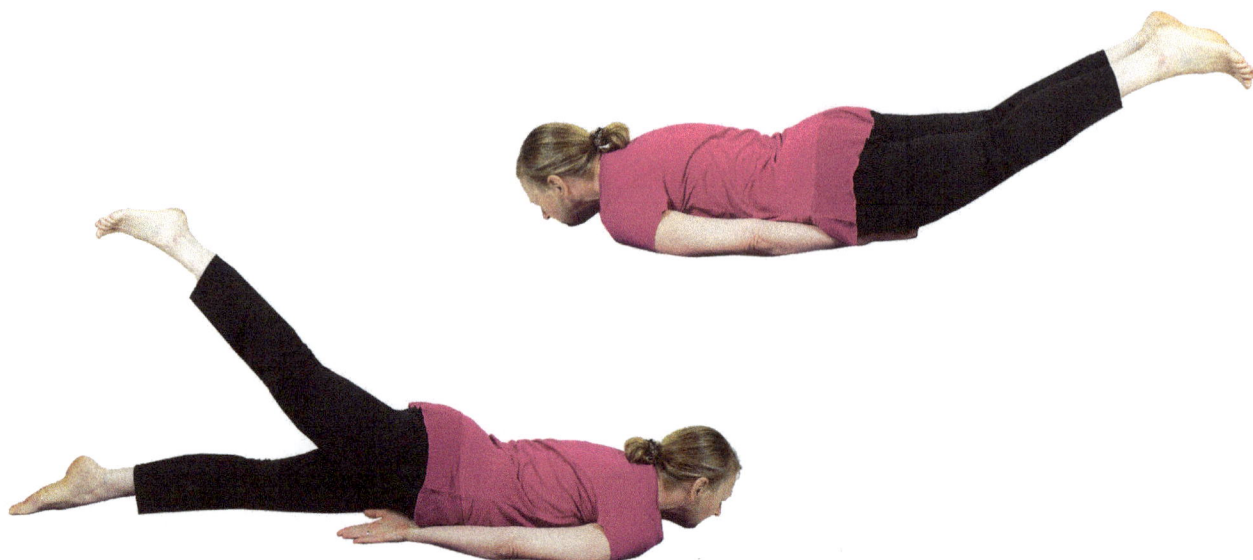

Start in Advasana. Place the forehead on the floor. Feet are hip-width apart, soles of the feet uppermost.

Place the hands under the thighs with the palms facing up or down.

Inhale, firm the abdomen and raise the right leg as high as possible behind you, keeping the leg straight and pointing the toes away from the body. Push down on the hands to help raise the leg. Use only the lower back muscles to do this rather than using the thigh muscles of the left leg.

Avoid twisting the pelvis.

Hold for the length of the inhaled breath, then exhale, relax the body and turn the head to one side.

Repeat to the other side.

Counterpose: This ⌒⌒ then ⌒⌒

Benefits: Works the back, spine and legs. Generally excellent for sciatica (but monitor how you feel after the practice to see if appropriate for you).

Start in Advasana. Place the forehead on the floor. Feet are hip-width apart, soles of the feet uppermost.

Make fists of the hands and roll the arms under the body. The fists lie in front of the hip bones.

Inhale, firm the abdomen and raise both legs as high as possible behind you, keeping the legs straight and pointing the toes away from the body. Push down on the fists and the arms and contract the lower back muscles to help raise the legs.

Hold for the length of the inhaled breath, then exhale, relax the body and turn the head to one side.

Repeat to the other side.

Modifications: ✿ Work with Ardha Salabhasana until the body is strong enough to do the full pose.

Counterpose: This ⌒⌒ then ⌒⌒

Benefits: Powerfully works the back, spine and legs.

Cautions: This is a strong asana requiring physical effort. Continue with Ardha Salabhasana if there are problems with the back, high blood pressure, hernia or heart conditions.

Salabhasana Variation –
Flying Locust Pose

Setu Bandhasana – *Bridge Pose*

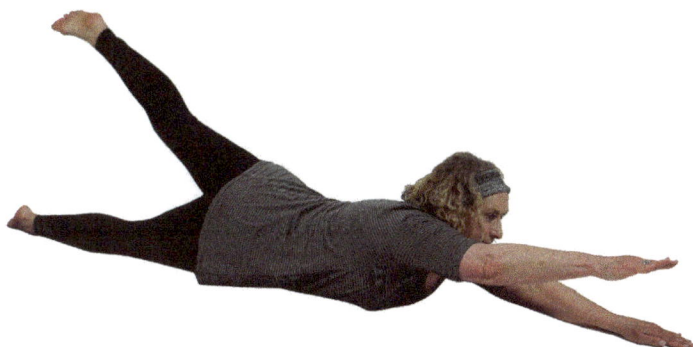

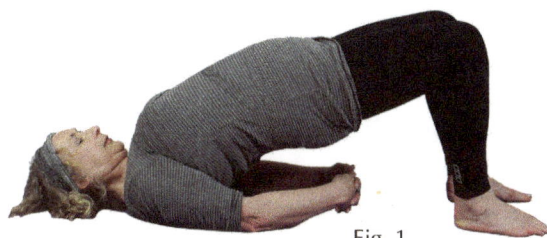

Fig. 1

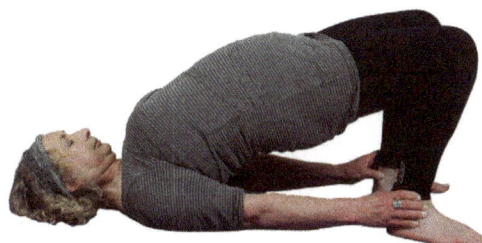

Fig. 2

This is an excellent practice to strengthen the back before practising the full Salabhasana (on previous page).

Start in Advasana. Place the chin on the floor. Feet are together and arms are stretched above the head, resting on the floor.

Stretch the right arm along the floor in front of you and stretch the left leg along the floor behind. Inhale, raise the right arm, left leg, head and chest off the floor. Hold the position for the length of the inhalation without straining.

Exhale, relax into Advasana once again.

Repeat the same movement to the left arm, right leg, head and chest.

Repeat up to five rounds.

Counterpose: This ⌒ then ⌒

Benefits: This asana strengthens weak and stiff backs and strengthens the back muscles. This is one of the few ways to give the body a diagonal stretch. It also develops concentration and coordination.

Lie on your back, knees bent, and draw the feet up near the buttocks, feet hip-width apart, the shins perpendicular to the floor.

Roll the whole of the arms under the body, from the shoulders to the hands. Interlock hands (Fig. 1). You can also roll the arms under the body and hold the backs of the ankles, although this stretch is out of reach for many people (Fig. 2).

Inhale, slowly raise the buttocks off the floor. Push down and out through the feet to raise the pelvis so that the thighs are parallel to the floor. Make sure the head and neck are lengthened on the floor by tucking in the neck.

To release, exhale and slowly lower to the floor.

Modification: ✿ As above, but keep arms alongside the body. Inhale, slowly lifting arms over the head to the floor behind. Exhale, slowly lower back to the floor.

Counterpose: This ⌒ then ⌒

Benefits: Beneficial for the digestive system, the spine, pelvis and legs, and stretches the upper back and neck. Works the lungs and opens the chest.

Cautions: Be careful if you have any back or neck problems. Modify.

Supta Pawanmuktasana
Stage 1 – *Leg Lock Pose*

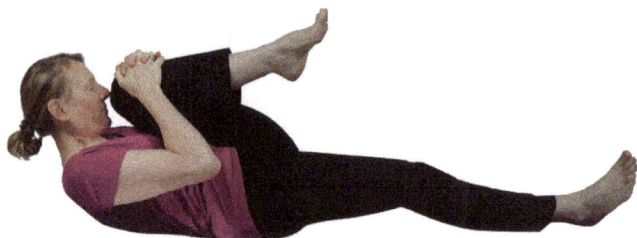

Stage 1

Supta Pawanmuktasana
Stage 2 – *Leg Lock Pose*

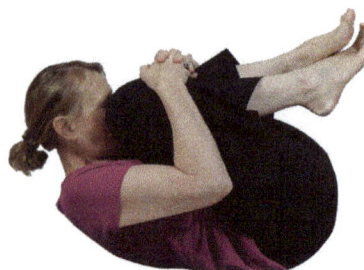

Stage 2

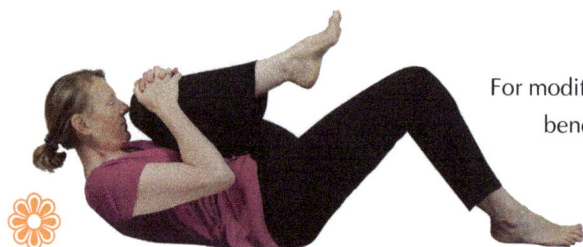

For modified version,
bend knee

Stage 1

Lie in the base position, flat on the back with the legs together and straight.

Bend the right knee and bring it to the chest. Wrap the hands around the shin just below the knee. The left leg stays in a straight line on the floor.

Inhale, lift the head and shoulders off the floor and try to bring the nose to the right knee. Try to hold this position for approximately the count of 3.

Then exhale, slowly lowering to the base position once again.

Let the body relax and do several more to this side, and then repeat the same number of times to the other side.

Modifications: ❁ If you have back problems, raise the left leg to semi-supine to ease the strain on the back. It is best to practise Stage 1 for some time before attempting Stage 2.

Benefits: Strengthens the lower back muscles and massages the abdomen and the digestive organs.

Cautions: Avoid if suffering from high blood pressure or serious back problems.

Stage 2

Lie in the base position. Bend the legs and bring both knees to the chest, and wrap the hands around the shins just below the knee.

Inhale and lift the head and shoulders off the floor. Try to bring the nose to the space between the knees. Hold the position for approximately the count of 3. Exhale and slowly lower to the base position once again.

Benefits: Strengthens the lower back muscles and massages the abdomen and the digestive organs.

Cautions: Avoid if suffering from high blood pressure or serious back problems.

It's not what happens but what you tell yourself that makes things awful, good or bad.

– Bernard Gunther

Pelvic Lifting

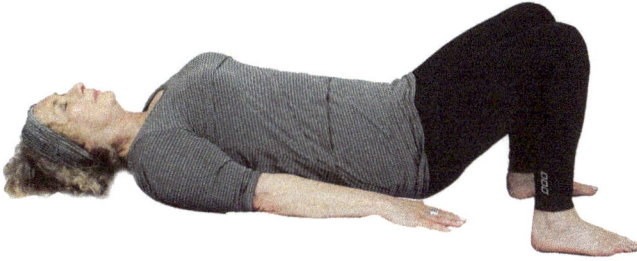

Supta Udarakarshanasana –
Sleeping Abdominal Stretch Pose

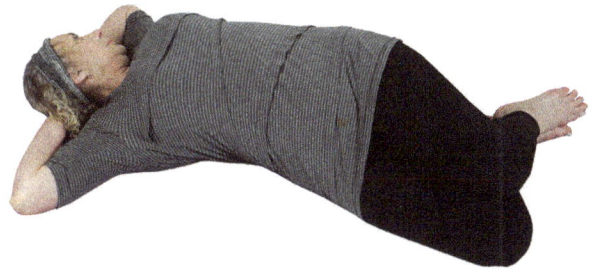

Lie in the base position, flat on the back with the legs together and straight.

Bend the knees bringing the feet up near the buttocks, feet flat on the floor and feet hip-width apart, shins vertical to the floor. Arms lie alongside the body, palms down.

Inhale, gently exaggerate the arch in the lower back and hold momentarily. Exhale, push the lower back into the floor. The buttocks will roll around but do not lift off the floor. Then keep repeating these movements, rolling gently from inhalation to exhalation.

Do not use force, it is a wave-like movement with the breath.

Benefits: This movement helps the muscles in this area to relax and brings flexibility and strength to this area. An excellent practice for this sometimes troublesome area of the lower back.

The snow goose need not bathe to make itself white, neither need you do anything but be yourself.

– Lao-Tzu

Lie in the base position, flat on the back with the legs together and straight.

Bend the knees, bringing the feet up near the buttocks, feet flat on the floor and together, shins vertical to the floor. Interlock the arms underneath the head.

Inhale, bring the knees to the floor on the right side, and turn to look at the elbow of the left arm.

Hold for a count of 3, then bring the head back to the centre, inhale and raise the legs to vertical. Exhale and take the knees to the floor on the left side, turn the head to look at the elbow of the right arm. Hold for the same count. Then keep practising, side to side.

Always bring the head back to the central position before raising the legs.

Modification: ❀ Stretch the arms out to the sides of the body at shoulder height, and turn to look at the right or left hand instead of the elbows.

Counterpose: 🐟

Benefits: Stretches the abdominal muscles and organs, improving digestion.

Cautions: Take care if you have lower back issues.

Adha Sarvangasana –
Half Shoulder Stand Pose

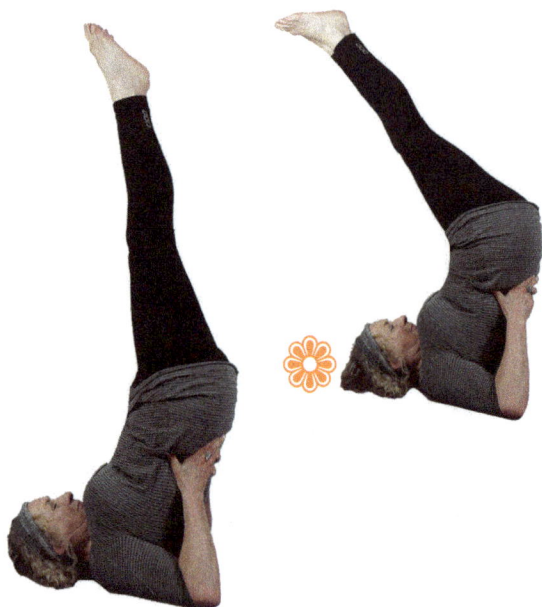

Vipareeta Karani Variation –
Legs up the Wall

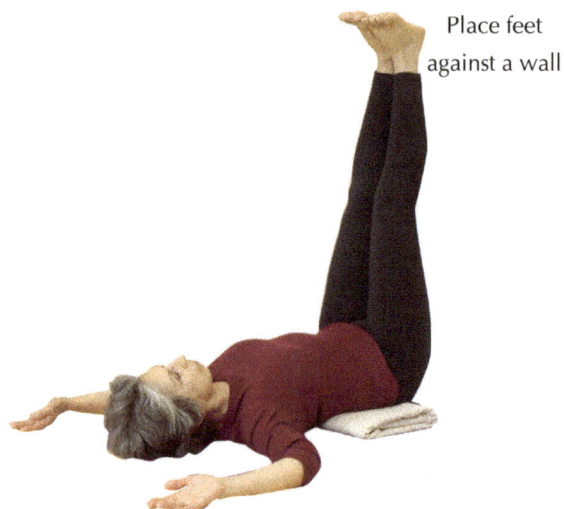

Place feet
against a wall

Lie flat on the back with the legs together and straight. Contract the abdominal muscles. Inhale, bring the knees to the chest and swing the pelvis off the floor moving the legs over the body towards the head. Support the body and back with your hands cupping the hip bones. The arms are close to the body with the elbows in line with the shoulders. Exhale then inhale and slowly raise the legs to the vertical position.

In the final position the weight of the body rests on the shoulders, neck and elbows, and the trunk is at a 45⁰ angle to the floor. Legs are as vertical as possible. The hands may slide further up the back for support. To release, bring the knees to the chest, support the back with your hands and roll down to the floor.

Modification: ✿ As shown above, allowing the legs to lean over the head, or adopt Vipareeta Karani Pose with legs up the wall (see adjoining column).

Counterpose: Matsyasana opposite page or

Benefits: Stimulates thyroid, parathyroid and thymus glands. Tones the legs, massages abdominal organs, drains stagnant blood and fluid, and improves circulation. It also relieves stress as the nervous system slows down.

Cautions: Avoid if there are problems with neck, spine, shoulders, heart, high blood pressure, thrombosis, thyroid disease, ear or eye problems.

This pose is an excellent substitute for the pose Adha Sarvangasana, with many of the same benefits.

Begin by sitting alongside a wall with the outside of one hip and shoulder against the wall and your hands behind you on the floor. Have a folded blanket at the ready.

Lean back on the hands, bring knees to the chest then swing and swivel the body around to lie at right angles to the wall, and extend the legs to vertical. Place your folded blanket under the hips and buttocks to give the back a further lift off the floor. Close the eyes and release deeply into the pose, surrendering to the stillness.

Benefits: The breathing becomes slower and deeper and the heart rate slows. This quietens the nervous system and the body feels rejuvenated. The internal organs are massaged. The effects of gravity on the circulatory system are reversed with the pelvis and legs raised higher than the heart and head, giving a rich supply of arterial blood to the head and glands of the upper body. Venous blood, which pools in the legs and abdomen, is drained.

Inversions restore the body's systems. They give vitality and bring one to a state of harmonious balance.

Halasana – *Plough Pose*

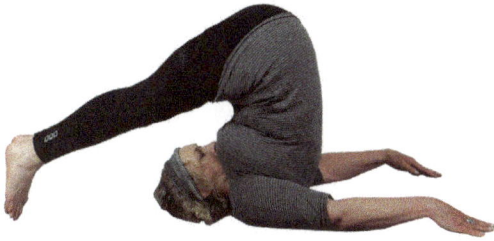

In the full pose toes touch the floor

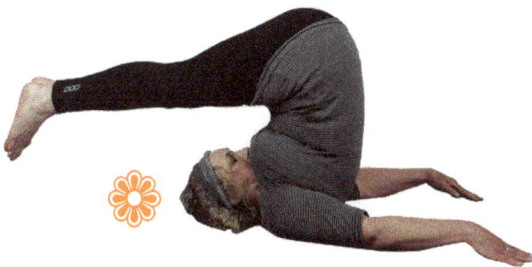

Come into Adha Sarvangasana (see previous page).

After a few deep breaths, firm the abdomen and work the hands towards the shoulder blades, and on an exhalation, extend straight legs from overhead to the floor behind. The toes come towards the floor, touching if possible. The spine remains straight, buttocks in line with the shoulders. The arms rest on the floor with the palms facing down. Breathe deeply.

To release, place the hands to support the back, bend the knees to the chest, and slowly roll back down to the floor near the buttocks, then extend the legs fully.

Modification: Gently stretch legs over head without placing toes on the floor, or practise Vipareeta Karani Pose (see previous page).

Counterpose: Matsyasana (opposite) or

Benefits: Massages internal organs, activates digestion, helps regulate thyroid/parathyroid and thymus glands, stretches neck, spine and hips. Improves liver and kidney functions, and overall circulation, particularly in the legs.

Cautions: Avoid if there are issues with the neck, shoulders, heart problems, high blood pressure, ear or eye problems. Not appropriate for breathing difficulties or problems with obesity. Avoid if lower back issues. Take care not to strain.

Matsyasana – *Fish Pose*

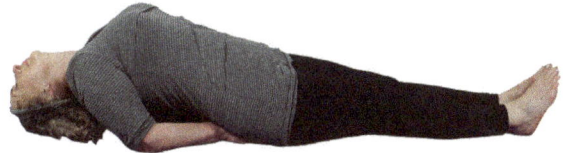

Matsyasana is commonly used as a counterpose for Adha Sarvangasana but is also a stand alone backward bend.

Place the lower arms underneath the body, palms facing down. From a lying position, prop up on the elbows and arch the spine. Inhale, and as the chest expands, lift the sternum, arch the spine backwards and slowly and gently lower the top of the head to the floor.

Exhale, and slowly ease the elbow outwards to allow the head better access to the floor. The weight is supported by the legs, buttocks, forearms and head. Make sure as little of the weight as possible is on the head.

To release, slide elbows out to release the back to the floor, bring the chin to the chest and rest flat on the floor.

Note: Traditionally in Matsyasana, the legs are placed in Lotus Pose.

Counterpose:

Benefits: Regulates thymus and thyroid glands. This pose also opens the chest encouraging deep respiration, and brings suppleness to the spine.

Cautions: Do not attempt this asana if there are any neck problems.

Adho Mukha Svanasana –
Downward Facing Dog Pose

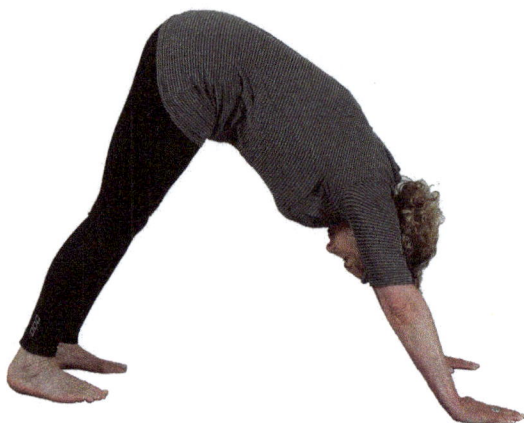

Ardha Adho Mukha Svanasana –
Half Downward Facing Dog Pose

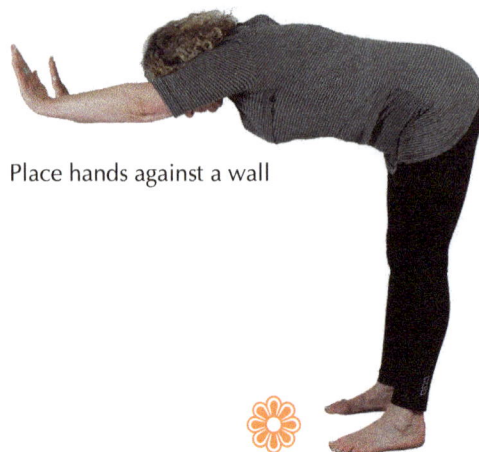

Place hands against a wall

Begin on all fours. Thighs are vertical to the floor, hands a little further forward than the shoulders. Spread the fingers with the middle finger pointing straight ahead. Tuck the toes under.

Inhale, engage the abdominal muscles and come up on the toes, lifting the buttocks towards the ceiling. Exhale, push back with the buttocks and lower the heels to the floor. Rotate the elbows and shoulders outwards. Move the chest towards the thighs and lengthen through the spine. Keep the head in line with the spine, ears alongside the arms.

To release, exhale and bring knees to the floor. Sit back on the heels to reverse the flow of blood to the head.

Modifications: If heels don't come to the floor, slowly and gently walk the feet up and down in a heel/toe action. Modify with Half Downward Facing Dog (see next column) if you have health problems.

Counterpose:

Benefits: Energises and stimulates the entire metabolism. Stretches the hamstrings, works the shoulders, improves blood flow and lymph, slows the breath and heart rate.

Cautions: Not appropriate for people with high blood pressure or eye conditions.

For people who cannot manage the full Downward Facing Dog due to health problems, this is an excellent alternative.

Place your hands against a wall, shoulder-width apart and at shoulder-height. Then step the feet back until they are perpendicular to the floor. Spread your fingers and push them against the wall, as if to push it away from you. Lower your head between the arms and lengthen out through the spine by pushing the buttocks away. Head, neck and spine are in a straight line.

You should feel a stretch in the hamstrings, and a stretch down the full length of the spine and across the shoulders and rib cage.

Benefits: Stretches the fingers, wrists, elbows, shoulders, rib cage, pelvis and backs of the thighs.

As human beings, our greatness lies not so much in being able to remake the world ... as in being able to remake ourselves.

– Mahatma Gandhi

Benefits of Asana

Forward stretching postures

These asanas always begin with a hinge-like folding movement at the hips (not the waist), so that the spine maintains its normal straight line. The whole of the body, from the heels to the back of the head, is stretched in these poses, and over time these asanas help the hip joints to become more flexible. The whole nervous system is revitalised, enhancing all the functions of the body. Circulation is improved and the endocrine glands and digestive system are also stimulated to work at their best. Forward bending poses are introverting and give us an opportunity to focus internally, which helps soothe and quieten the mind. In these asanas we must be even more mindful of our limitations. *Caution*: If you have back issues, do these asanas with great care.

Back arching postures

In our daily routines, we rarely arch backwards. These asanas open the chest wide, enhancing our sense of confidence. They are stimulating and extroverting. They also strengthen the back and bring flexibility to the spine. They facilitate deep breathing, relieve stiffness of the neck, shoulder blades and joints. The digestive system is stimulated, and the adrenal glands, kidneys and urinary tract are also influenced positively. The practices can help to correct postural problems and muscular imbalances in the spine.

Balance postures

In these postures, mind and body must work as one to achieve the pose. Balance poses are not static as they are influenced by the movement of the breath and require constant micro adjustments. Over time, these postures help to improve our concentration and balance at physical, as well as emotional and mental levels. They help balance the nervous system and relieve stress and anxiety, bringing about a sense of peace and harmony.
Practice tip: It helps concentration to focus on a point in front of you called a 'drishti point'. Gaze softly at this point and it will help you maintain your balance.

Side stretching postures

Side stretching strengthens the muscles and joints of the whole body. Lateral spinal movement is easily lost as we age and should be practised on a regular basis. This movement can release backache and neck stiffness, and generally improves our suppleness of movement. Side stretching also massages the abdominal organs at the same time, expanding the chest on alternate sides. The hip joints and leg muscles are also strongly worked.

Twisting postures

Spinal twisting can improve spinal flexibility, which in turn can free trapped, compressed nerves and contracted muscles, allowing energy to flow to all parts of the body. During twisting, the abdominal organs receive a gentle massage through the squeezing activity of the twists. These asanas tone the nervous system by activating and stimulating the nerve plexuses in the abdomen, as well as the spinal nerves. Twists also increase the pranic flow, nourishing the abdominal organs and rejuvenating the tissues generally. Twisting also helps to reset the spine and is often done at the end of an asana session. These asanas have a powerful effect on our overall health and vitality.

Inverted postures

In these asanas, the body is required to maintain balance whilst working against the pull of gravity. In all cases, the head is below the heart, which allows a rich supply of blood to flow to the head, energising and stimulating the brain and nourishing the neurons. Inverted asanas improve the flow of blood and lymph, and are revitalising. All inverted poses affect the pituitary gland which in turn benefits all the endocrine glands. This has a positive effect on the entire metabolism. The breath becomes slow and deep, encouraging correct breathing habits, and the heart rate slows down.

Surya Namaskara – *Salute to the Sun*

Surya Namaskara is a popular yoga practice that is done dynamically, moving from one posture to the next with concentration on the breath. This practice, if done daily, can very quickly bring flexibility and strength to the body, as well as tone all the joints, muscles and internal organs.

The 12 positions of Surya Namaskara relate to the 12 solar phases of the year.

Surya Namaskara also comprises several practices in one, including pranayama (as each movement is done to a specific breath), mantra yoga (as each pose has a specific mantra attached to it), and if done with the eyes closed, the rhythmic movements can induce a meditative state.

The dynamic nature of this group of asanas also draws a high level of prana (life force) into the body. The practice stimulates and regulates pingala nadi (the solar nadi) which brings balance to the energy system of the mind and body.

Surya Namaskara is an excellent practice to begin the day with, ideally facing east as the sun rises, although any time of the day is appropriate.

To be in the spirit of this ancient practice, take some time to stand in Tadasana with the eyes closed, and become aware of your whole physical body from head to toes. Feel into your body, slowly releasing any tension or tightness. Feel the body slowly start to relax and soften. Then bring to your awareness an image of the blazing sun and feel the energy of the sun flooding through your body and mind, energising your body to prepare for this flowing yoga dance.

If you have not practised this before, it is best to start slowly with 2 or 3 full rounds. The 12 positions have to be completed twice to complete 1 full found. In the first round, the right foot is stepped backwards in position 4, and the the left is stepped forward in position 9. In the second cycle, the left is stepped backward in position 4 and the right is stepped forward in position 9.

Modifications: ✺ The modified version is given overleaf.

Counterpose: ⟶ Lie in Savasana until the heart rate and breath return to normal.

Benefits: This practice stimulates and balances every system in the body.

Cautions: Must be practised on an empty stomach. Do some limbering before commencing (see the limbering section). Because of the dynamic nature of this practice, it is not appropriate for people with heart conditions, history of a stroke or high blood pressure, or for people with eye conditions such as glaucoma or a history of detached retina.

People with back conditions should consult a medical practitioner before introducing Surya Namaskara to their yoga routine.

Surya Mantras

There is a Surya Mantra for each of the positions of the practice.

1. *Om Mitraya Namaha*
2. *Om Ravaye Namaha*
3. *Om Suryaya Namaha*
4. *Om Bhanave Namaha*
5. *Om Khagaya Namaha*
6. *Om Pushne Namaha*
7. *Om Hiranya Garbhaya Namaha*
8. *Om Marichaye Namaha*
9. *Om Adityaya Namaha*
10. *Om Savitre Namaha*
11. *Om Arkaya Namaha*
12. *Om Bhaskaraya Namaha*

There is also a Beeja Mantra for each of the positions.

1. *Om Hraam*
2. *Om Hreem*
3. *Om Hroom*
4. *Om Hraim*
5. *Om Hraum*
6. *Om Hrah*
7. *Om Hraam*
8. *Om Hreem*
9. *Om Hroom*
10. *Om Hraim*
11. *Om Hraum*
12. *Om Hrah*

Surya Namaskara
Salute to the Sun

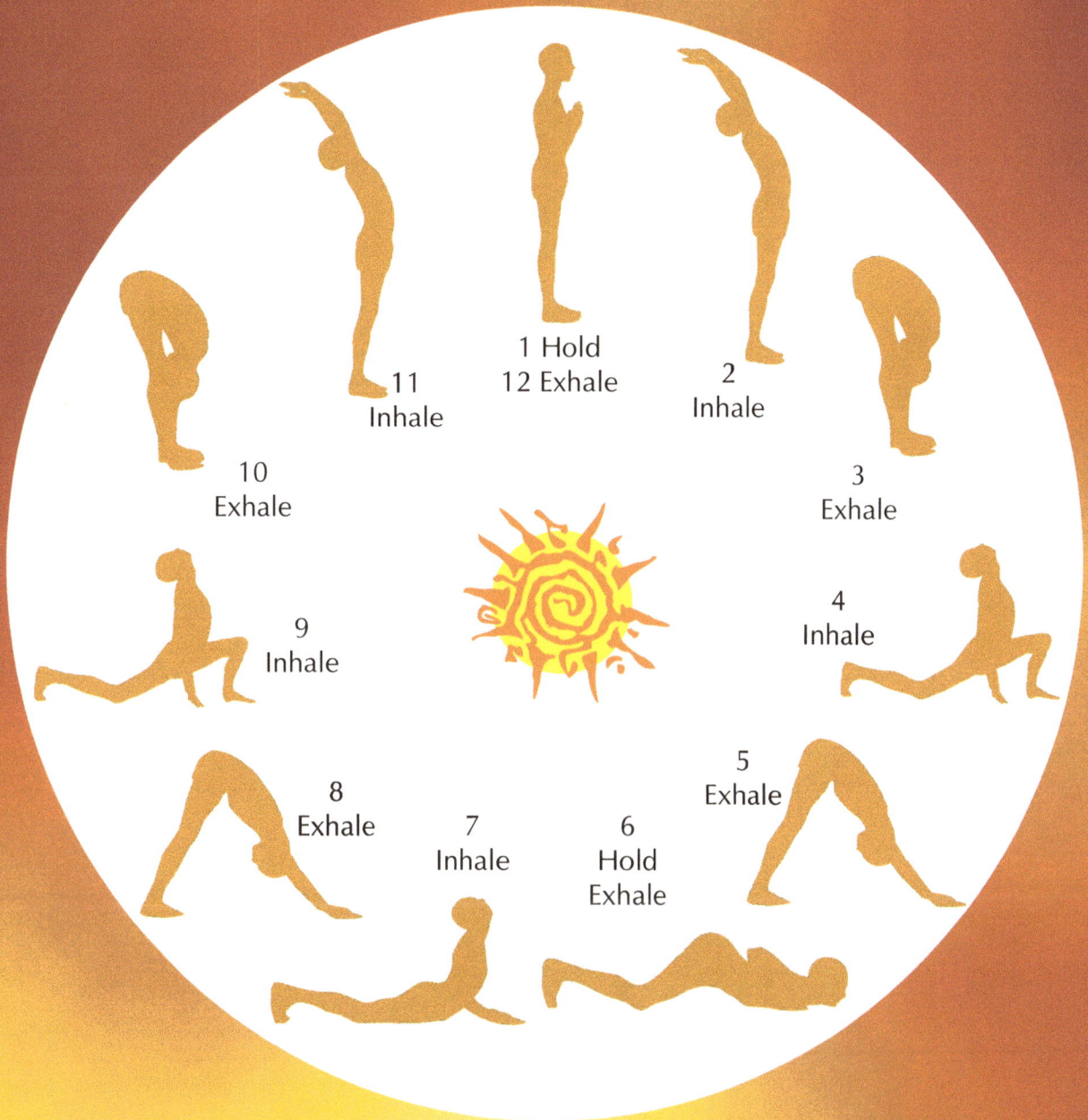

1 Hold
12 Exhale

11 Inhale

2 Inhale

10 Exhale

3 Exhale

9 Inhale

4 Inhale

8 Exhale

5 Exhale

7 Inhale

6 Hold Exhale

The 12 positions are to be practised twice to complete one full found.

Round 1: the right foot is stepped back in position 4, and the the left is stepped forward in position 9.

Round 2: the left is stepped back in position 4 and the right is stepped forward in position 9.

Surya Namaskara
Salute to the Sun (Modified)

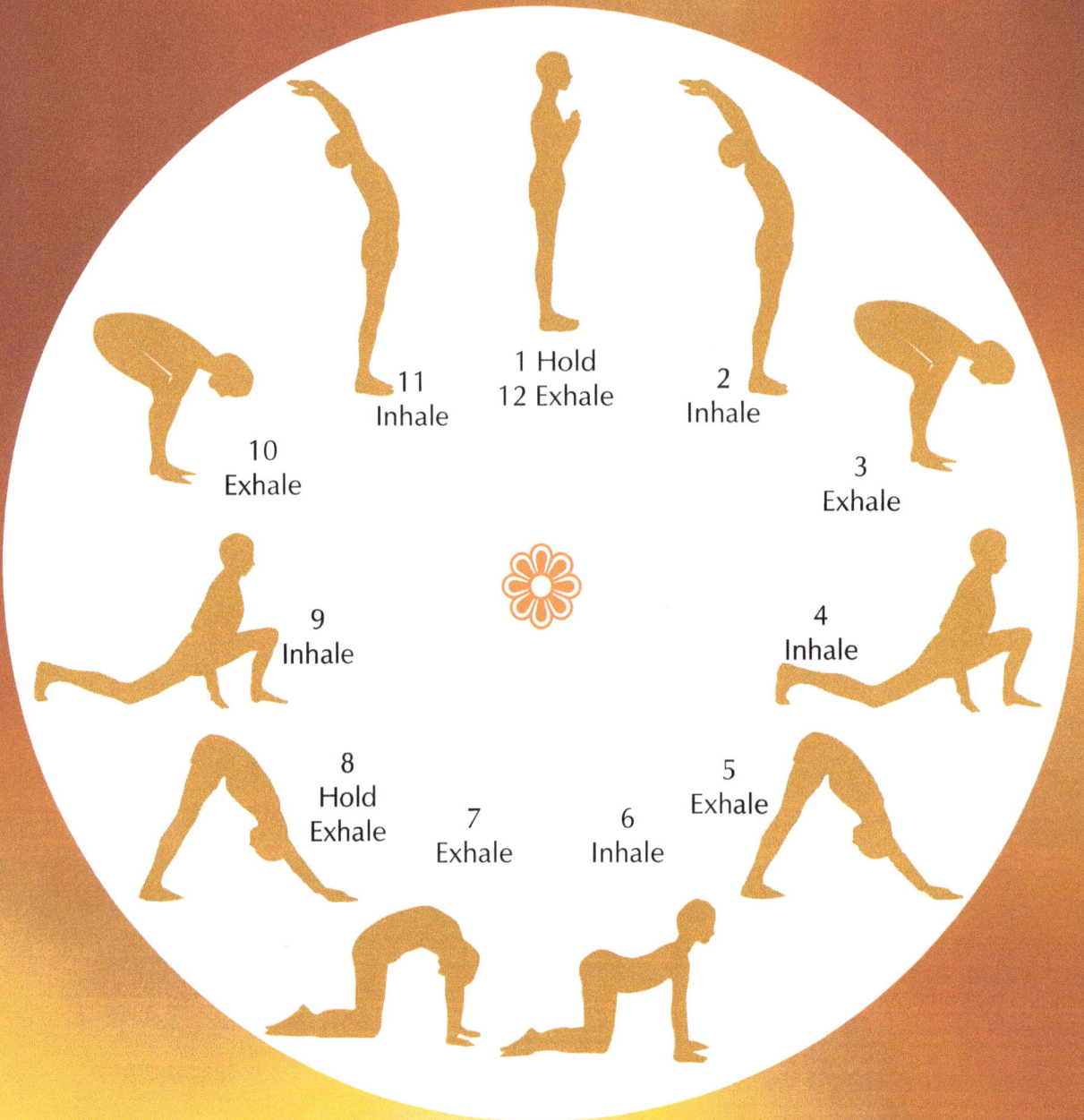

11 Inhale

1 Hold
12 Exhale

2 Inhale

10 Exhale

3 Exhale

9 Inhale

4 Inhale

8 Hold Exhale

7 Exhale

6 Inhale

5 Exhale

The 12 positions have to be completed twice to complete one full found.

Round 1: the right foot is stepped back in position 4, and the the left is stepped forward in position 9.

Round 2: the left is stepped back in position 4 and the right is stepped forward in position 9.

Chandra Namaskara
Salute to the Moon

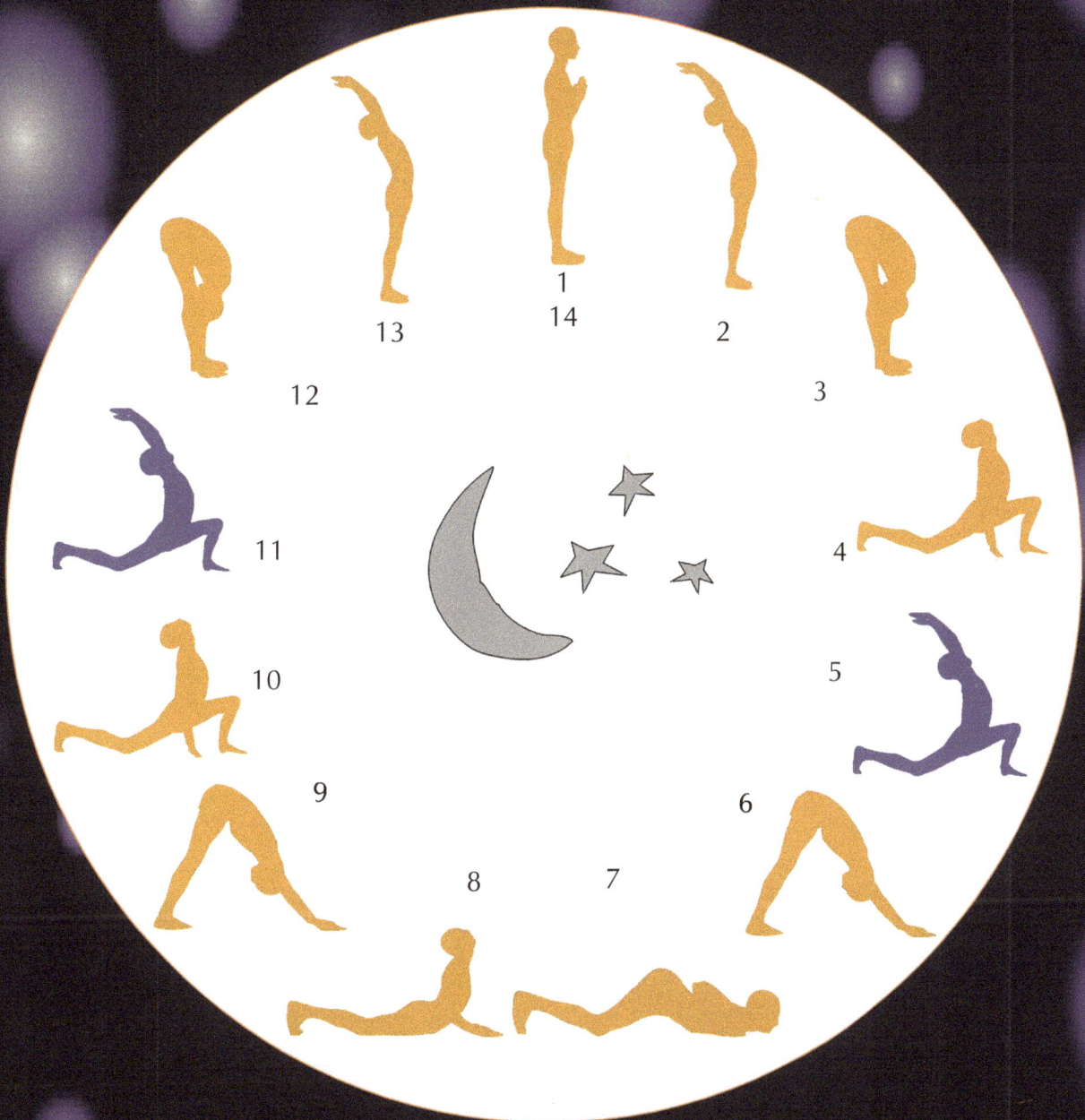

1

14

13

2

12

3

11

4

10

5

9

6

8

7

Just as the moon reflects the light of the sun, the practice of Chandra Namaskara reflects that of Surya Namaskara except Ardha Chandrasana Pose (5 & 11) has been included. This asana requires balance and concentration, adding another dimension to the practice.

Breathing: unlike the dynamic practice of Surya Namaskara, Ardha Chandrasana is a contemplative practice, so several breaths should be taken at each position.

Putting It All Together

❖ Start by relaxing the body. Lie on the floor in Shavasana with eyes closed. Focus on the breath.

❖ Then start with movements to limber the body and gently work through the joints.

❖ After limbering start sequencing the postures. Do standing asanas together, and likewise for sitting, prone and supine, making a smooth transition from one asana to the next with minimal disruption between each pose. (Draw up a practice plan – see opposite page.)

❖ Work mindfully with full awareness of the body, breath, joints and muscles.

❖ Maintain alignment rather than forcing into the pose, and move just a little past your comfort zone.

❖ Choose to work through forward stretching, backward stretching, side stretching, twisting, inversions, and balances.

❖ Always counterpose the strong asanas as shown.

❖ You can choose to do the asanas statically or dynamically. When done statically, they are performed with little movement, holding the body in position for some time, focusing on the body and breath. The internal organs are gently massaged, the muscles, ligament and tendons are stretched, and the nervous system relaxes.

If working dynamically, the body moves energetically from one position to the next, increasing the heart rate, working on fitness, releasing energy blocks, strengthening the muscles, lungs and digestive system. Surya Namaskara (p. 52) is an example of working dynamically.

❖ After asana, pranayama practice (breath work) is recommended, followed by relaxation or meditation.

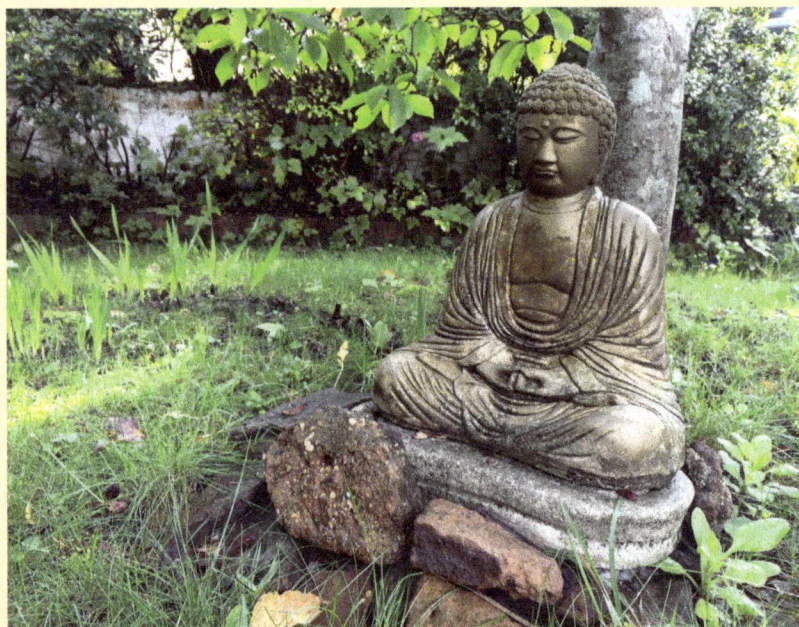

Home Practice

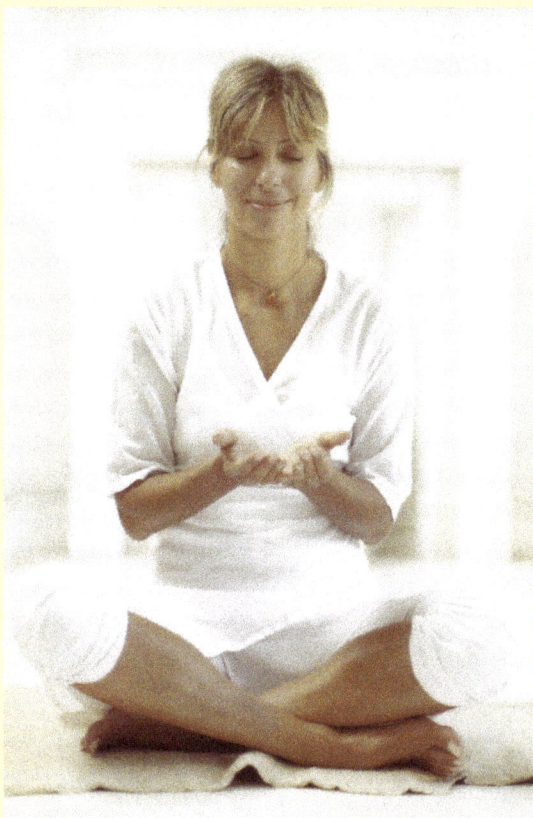

In order for your home practice to flow, it is beneficial to write up a yoga sequence beforehand. This way you don't have to stop the flow of your practice to think of what to do next.

An easy way to do this is with stick figures. It is true that 'a picture speaks a thousand words'. You only have to glance at your practice sheet to know what to do next, rather than read instructions.

Stick figures are very easy to draw. Just start with the head and spine; a dot or line for the nose shows which direction the head is facing. Add arms and legs, and whatever other detail you find helpful. If there is an asana you just can't manage to capture as a stick figure, make up your own symbol to denote this asana.

A few examples follow. I am sure you will know which asanas they represent.

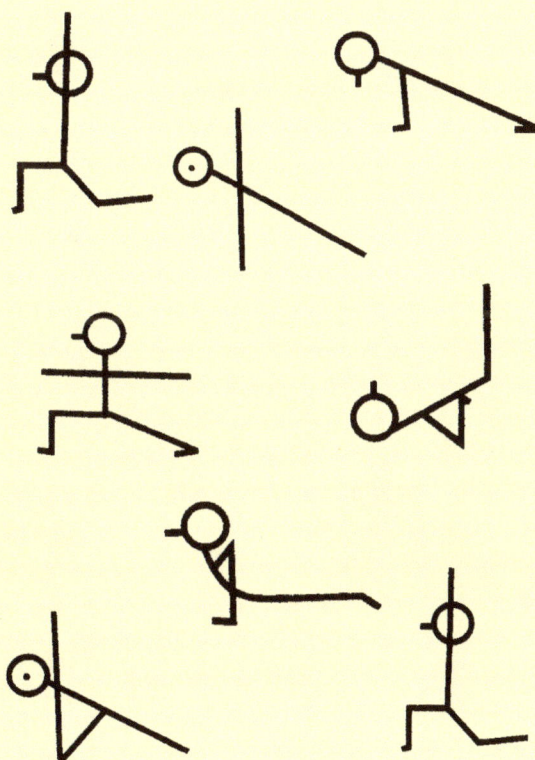

Attending a yoga class once a week is excellent, but adding a home practice is even better. It can do wonders for your flexibility and strength.

Any time of day is suitable for practising yoga except immediately after meals. It is generally felt that early morning is best. However, one is less flexible in the morning, so it is important to do limbering beforehand. As the day progresses the body becomes more flexible.

It can be difficult sometimes to make a commitment to doing yoga practice on a regular basis. It helps if you have a place where you can leave your mat on the floor, as this can work as a constant reminder and it is one less thing to do before starting your practice. If you are disinclined to make a start, just sit on the mat and begin to do some gentle movements of the joints and before you know it, your body will want to do more.

Limbering the Body

Before you begin yoga asana, it is important to do preparatory practices to work the major joints and relax the muscles. As you focus on limbering and stretching the body, releasing tension and stress, the mind starts to relax as it lets go of restrictive thinking; then you can move more fluidly through the asanas.

This 'warming up' of the body encourages the synovial fluid to lubricate the joints, helping them to work more efficiently. Warming the muscles by stretching and contracting allows them to work through the asana with less risk of injury; it also brings *prana* (life force) which also gives greater energy for the practice.

The following are just a few of the limbering possibilities. Limbering can start from supine, sitting or standing positions.

Limbering from Supine (L–R)

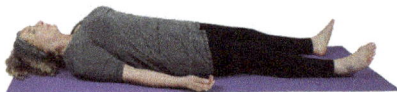

Lie in *Shavasana* for several minutes, observing the breath.

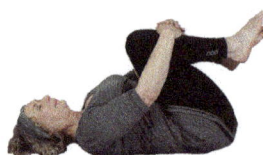

Bring knees to chest, hands around shins, and gently rock from side to side for a few minutes.

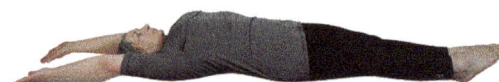

Inhale, lift arms over head, point toes and fingers, and stretch through the body (2 rounds).

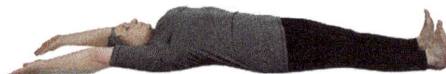

Inhale, lift arms over head, flex toes towards the trunk and stretch through the body (2 rounds).

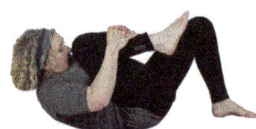

Legs bent at the knees. Bend right knee and wrap hands around shin, drawing the knee into the chest. Inhale, then exhale, bring nosetip towards the knee. Hold for count of 3 (5 rounds). Repeat to other side.

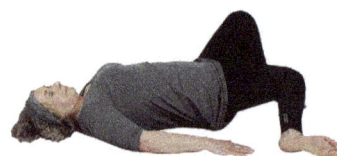

Legs bent at the knees, with feet out to the edge of the mat. Inhale, then exhale and drop right knee inwards to the floor alongside the left ankle. Inhale, return. Repeat to the other side (10 rounds each side).

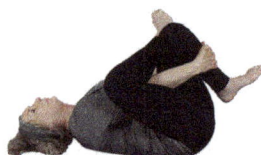

Legs bent at the knees. Draw right knee to chest, swing knee out to the side, placing right foot on left thigh. Lift left leg slightly, reach up and place hands around the left thigh, then bring head back to the floor. Hold for a count of 20, then repeat to the other side.

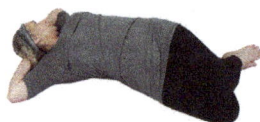

Legs bent at the knees, with feet together. Hands interlocked under head. Inhale, then exhale and bring knees to the floor on right side, simultaneously turning head to look at left elbow. Inhale, return head and knees to centre. Repeat to the other side (10 rounds).

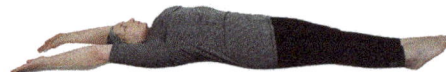

Have feet hip-width apart and relaxed out to the sides. Inhale, slowly raise arms overhead as you peel the trunk up from the floor. Exhale, slowly release back to the floor (5 rounds).
Note: Avoid this practice if you have any back issues.

Limbering from Sitting (L–R)

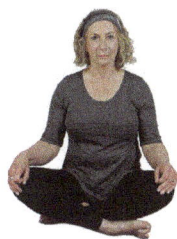

Sit for several minutes observing the breath.

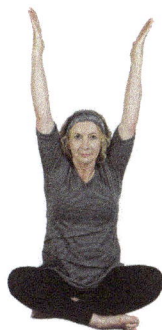

Inhale and float arms out to the side and over the head (to a count of 4), then exhale and float arms back down (to a count of 4).

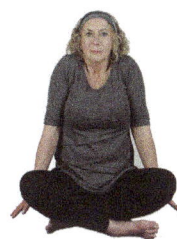

Inhale and raise the shoulders up to the ears, hold, then exhale with a loud 'haaaa' as you release the shoulders. Do several times.

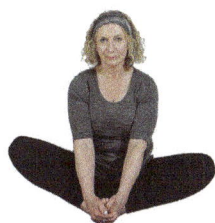

With a straight back, draw the soles of feet together and hands around feet. Butterfly (flap) both the knees dynamically up and down (20 times).

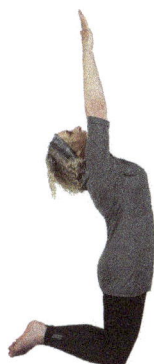

Sit on the heels to start, then come up onto knees, inhale and stretch arms overhead, arch back (keeping both thighs vertical). Exhale, and lower to the starting position (6 rounds).

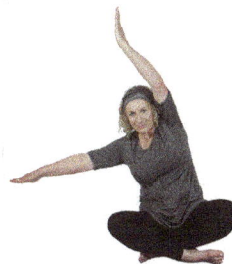

Stretch the right arm out to side. Inhale, stretch left arm overhead vertically, exhale bend and stretch left arm alongside ear. Stretch right arm to extend the movement. Breathe freely and count to 10, holding the stretch. Repeat to the other side.

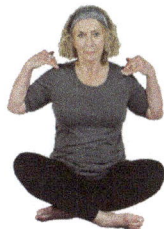

Fingertips on shoulders, inhale and bring elbows to touch in front, swing them up and around in a circular movement 10 times. Inhale upswing – exhale downswing. Then reverse direction for 10 rounds.

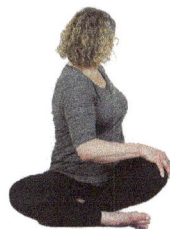

Sit in an easy pose. Place right hand on left knee, and left hand at the base of spine. Inhale, stretch up tall, exhale, twist the head and upper trunk to look over the left shoulder. Hold, then inhale and return to centre. Practise 4 times to the left, then switch hands and do 4 times to the right.

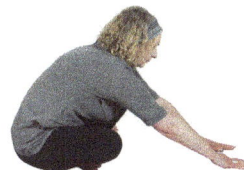

Sit in an easy pose. Place hands on the floor in front. Keeping back straight, slowly move hands forward until you reach your limit. Hold for a count of 10, breathing freely.

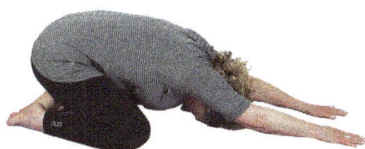

Sit on heels. Fold forward, forehead to floor. Stretch arms to front and walk fingers away from the body, stretching through the spine (1-2 rounds). Relax the whole body.

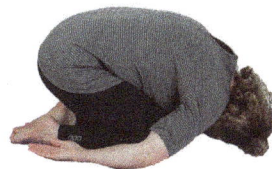

Sit on heels. Fold forward, bringing forehead to floor. Keep arms alongside body, palms face upwards. Breathe freely. Hold for a few minutes and internalise your awareness. Relax the whole body.

Limbering from Standing (L–R)

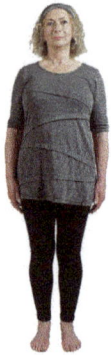

Stand in Tadasana for a few minutes and observe the breath.

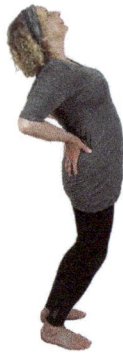

Stand in Tadasana. Spread hands across lower back, inhale, and on exhale, arch back, bending knees. Inhale, return to Tadasana.

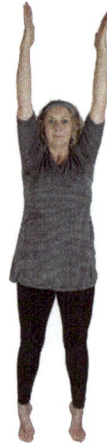

Stand in Tadasana. Inhale and float arms out to the side and over the head, at the same time coming up on the toes. Hold for the length of the inhalation. Then exhale, floating arms back down to the sides (5 rounds).

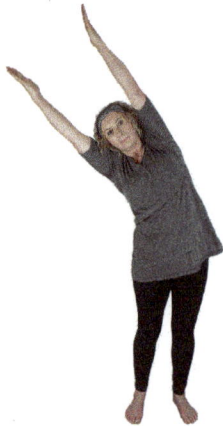

Stand in Tadasana. Inhale as you float arms out to the side and over the head, exhale and bend to the right side, keeping arms straight. Inhale, return to Tadasana, exhale and repeat to the other side (5 rounds).

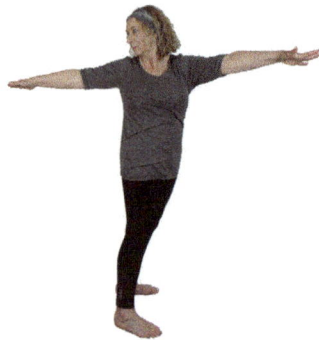

Stand in Tadasana, feet hip-width apart, toes turned inwards. Inhale, float arms up to shoulder height, and begin to wrap arms to the sides. Breathe freely. Eyes follow the movement of the arms. Practise a few rounds, allowing the body to let go into the movement.

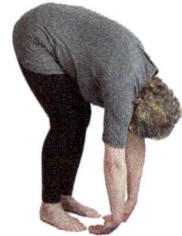

In Tadasana, inhale, bring chin to chest, exhale, slowly roll forward, knees bent if hamstrings tight. Let body release and relax, dangling forward breathing freely. Bend the knees, roll back up into Tadasana.

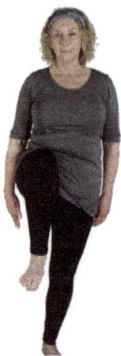

Stand in Tadasana. Keeping the back straight, inhale, bend the leg and raise the right knee as high as possible. Exhale, return the foot to the floor. Repeat from side to side as if marching on the spot.

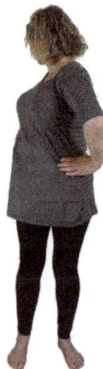

Stand in Tadasana. Hands on hips, slowly rotate the body as far as you can to the right then back to centre, and to the left (10 rounds).

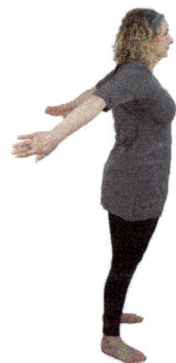

Stand in Tadasana. Swing arms to shoulder height to the front and then backwards as far as you can, lifting the shoulders as you swing back and forth. Breathe freely throughout. Practise a few rounds, allowing the body to let go into the movement.

Limbering Joints (L–R)

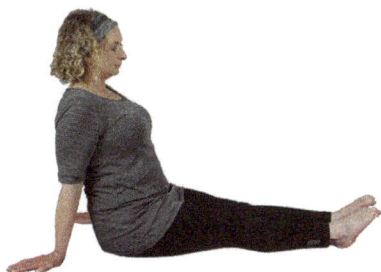

Lean back on hands, legs straight, bend toes forward on inhalation and backwards on exhalation.
(10 rounds).

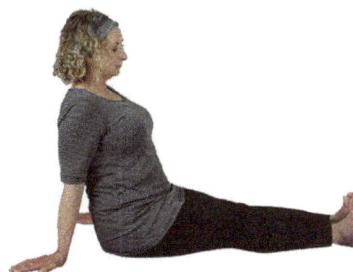

Lean back on hands, legs straight, Rotate ankles 10 times in one direction then 10 times in opposite direction.

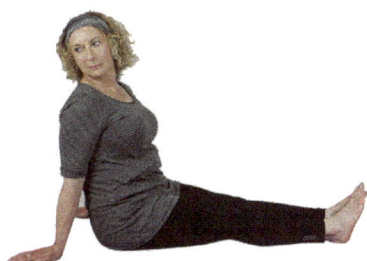

Sit upright with legs straight, inhale, then exhale turn the head as far as you can to the right, exhale back to the centre. Repeat to the other side (4 times to each side).

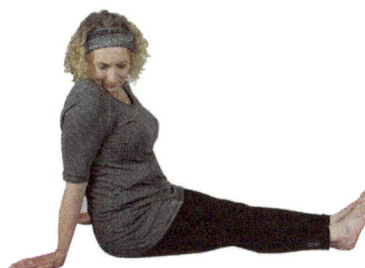

Bring chin to the chest and let the head dangle freely under its own weight for a slow count of 10, then pendulum swing the head gently across the front of the body from right shoulder to left. Take care not to strain.

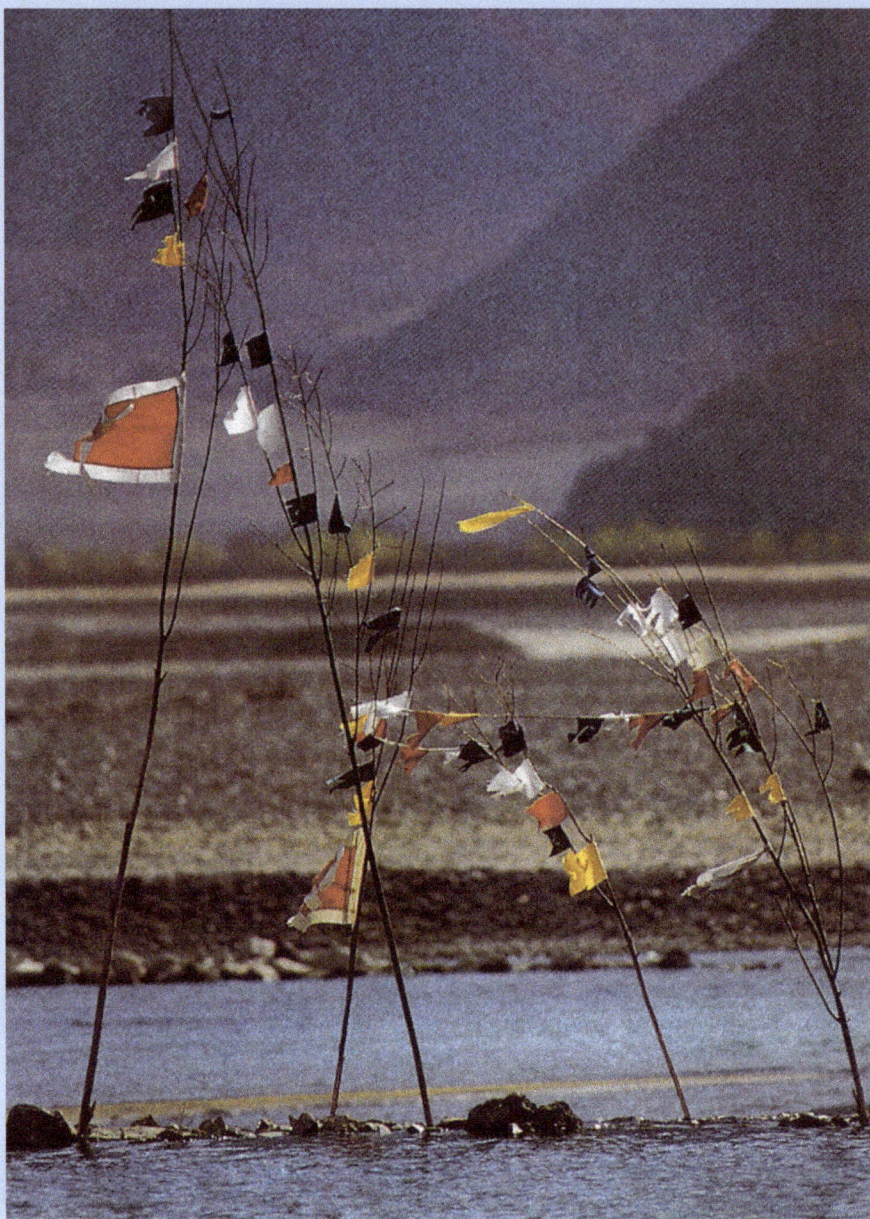

Pranayama

Breath Control

Free your breath, free your mind

Pranayama Overview

Prana is the life force or energy, as it permeates every living thing. We can absorb prana through the food we eat, through the water we drink, through the sunshine on our skin and through the air we breathe. Breathing gives the body life, and every one of the trillions of cells in our body requires oxygen to survive and be healthy.

The practice of pranayama gives us control over our breathing to aid the extension, expansion and assimilation of the life force through breathing techniques.

The breath holds the body and mind together, and once we know the correct way to breathe, we can influence in a positive way all the systems of the body, and control stress levels and our emotional health.

But before starting pranayama practice it is important to understand the mechanics of breathing and to learn how to breathe correctly. To be able to access good breathing habits, we need to understand a little of the anatomy and mechanics of breathing.

The mechanics of breathing

We have three choices regarding the muscles we use for breathing:

Clavicular: Breathing into the upper lobes of the lungs, which only happens with extreme exertion when the rest of the lungs are fully ventilated or when airways are constricted by illness (e.g., asthma).

Thoracic: Occurs in the middle of the chest (i.e., chest breathing). This breathing is mostly active after physical exertion but under normal circumstances, when the ribs simply move with inhalation and exhalation.

Diaphragmatic (abdominal): When the breath is inhaled right down to the lower lobes of the lungs. This is the correct breathing technique as it: *'. . . causes equal expansion of the alveoli, improves lymphatic draining, and massages the organs that lie in the pelvic cavity beneath it. It also benefits the cardiac functions and coronary supply and improves oxygenation of the blood and circulation'.*[1]

Elements of clavicular and thoracic breathing are part of normal breathing, but the diaphragm is the muscle best suited for expanding the lungs. However, when the body is stressed, the diaphragm locks. Breathing then becomes more rapid, and shallow breaths are taken in the chest region, which in turn arouses the sympathetic nervous system – this is the 'fight or flight' response. Restrictive clothing and poor posture has the same effect.

Because of the stresses in every day life, many people are locked into these bad breathing habits, namely chest breathing, which causes the heart rate to increase and the blood pressure to rise.

Prana is the life-force which permeates both the individual as well as the universe at all levels. It is at once physical, sexual, mental, intellectual, spiritual, and cosmic. Prana, the breath, and the mind are inextricably linked to each other.

– BKS Iyengar

[1] *Asana Pranayama Mudra Bandha* by Swami Satyananda Saraswati (published by Yoga Publications Trust, Munger, India)

PRANAYAMA CONTENTS

Pranayama (yogic breathing) is a vast subject covering the science of prana (vital energy) and the many practices that aim to increase this prana within the body and mind.

This is by no means the full range of pranayama practices. The ones offered here are those commonly practised in most yoga traditions and are well within the reach of mature age yoga practitioners.

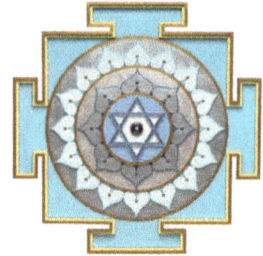

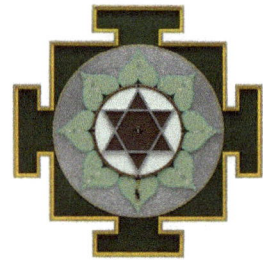

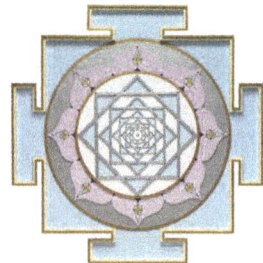

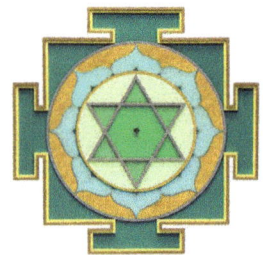

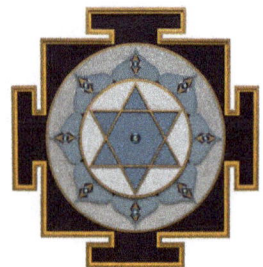

Diaphragmatic (Abdominal) Breathing

Inhalation

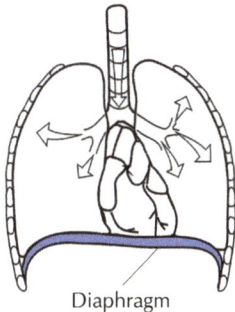

Diaphragm

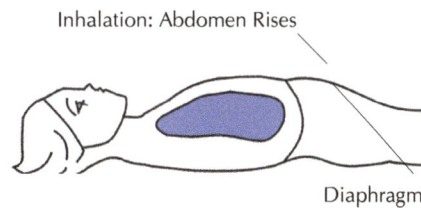

Inhalation: Abdomen Rises

Diaphragm

Exhalation

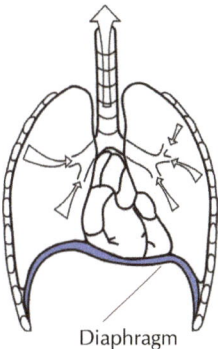

Diaphragm

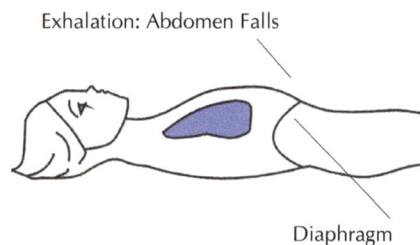

Exhalation: Abdomen Falls

Diaphragm

The diaphragm is a dome-shaped sheet of muscle that lies horizontally inside the body, dividing the body into the chest cavity (containing the heart and lungs) and the pelvic cavity (containing the organs of digestion, assimilation, elimination and reproduction).

When we inhale, the lungs expand and pull the diaphragm downwards into the pelvic cavity. When this happens, the abdominal organs are compressed downwards, pushing the abdomen outwards. When we exhale, the lungs shrink and the diaphragm relaxes and moves back up into the chest cavity and the abdomen contracts.

So when breathing is relaxed, the diaphragm moves with ease. If the body is stressed, the diaphragm locks up and the breath becomes short and shallow in the chest.

Poor breathing habits can leave the body low on oxygen which impedes the removal of waste matter from the body, so that the body retains these toxins and the whole system is basically starved of energy.

The diagrams above show how the diaphragm moves on inhalation and exhalation and how the abdomen rises and falls with this movement.

As you continue on the path of yoga, diaphragmatic breathing will serve as a foundation for many other practices.

And when fears seem overwhelming in the course of daily living, you will have an internal friend to comfort your mind.

All in all, as you improve the quality of your breathing, you will improve the quality of your life.

– Rolf Sovik
(President & Director, Himalayan Institute)

Regulate the breathing, and thereby control the mind.

– B.K.S. Iyengar

1. How to practise diaphragmatic (abdominal) breathing

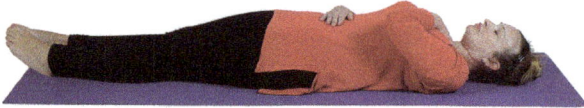

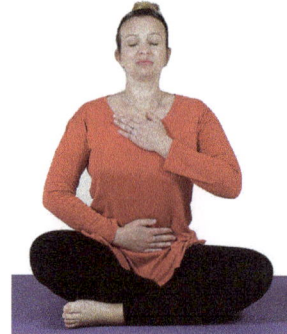

Lie in Shavasana and feel the body relaxing. Then focus the awareness on the breath and breathe naturally. When you feel completely relaxed and your breathing is natural, place the right hand on the abdomen and the left hand over the centre of the chest.

On the inhalation, draw the breath right down into the lower lobes of the lungs; the right hand will rise and on the exhalation the right hand will fall. The left hand will not move at all.

When lying down, it is easy to detect if you are breathing diaphragmatically. When sitting, if you are breathing in a relaxed diaphragmatic way, the breath no longer feels the same as when lying down. Now the inhalation still expands the abdomen but the movement is not as pronounced, and there is also some expansion of the sides of the rib cage.

Do not exaggerate the breath, it should be natural and automatic.
You are not the breather, the body breathes and you are the silent witness of the breath.

2. Modified Crocodile Pose trains the body to breathe diaphragmatically

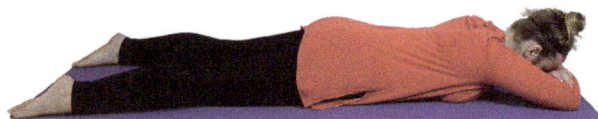

A wonderful way to observe the diaphragmatic breath and train the body to breathe in this way, is to practise the Crocodile Pose.

Lie prone on your stomach, with your forehead resting on your folded arms, hands reaching the opposite elbows. Extend the feet to the sides of your mat (wider than hip-width apart) with the heels turned inwards. The shoulders and upper chest will be elevated off the floor.

In this way, you immobilise the chest and shoulders and this trains you to breathe diaphragmatically and even strengthens the diaphragm.

You do not have to control the breath, it will find its own pace and rhythm.

On the inhalation, feel the breath moving into the lower back and the sides of the ribcage, and feel the ribs expand laterally. Also feel the abdomen working against resistance as it is pressed against the floor. This is an excellent feedback for diaphragmatic breath training.

Whenever you feel tension building in your body, lie for several minutes in Crocodile Pose. Your breath will become extremely relaxed, and it will help you gain control of your breath and to release pent-up tension.

The Full Yogic Breath

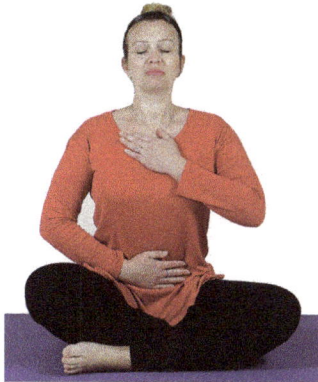

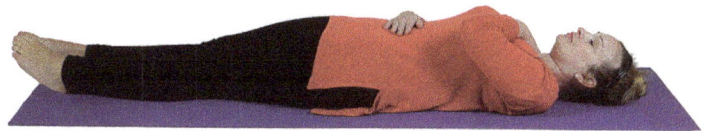

The full yogic breath is not practised continually. This breathing technique is used to gain control over our breathing (i.e., re-boot the system) or to correct poor breathing habits.

Full yogic breathing maximises the inhalation and exhalation and therefore increases lung ventilation. It is an excellent practice to calm the mind, as it releases endorphins.

Start sitting or lying with one hand on the belly and one on the chest to help track the movement of the breath. Start to breathe in a long, smooth relaxed way through the following sequence.

Inhale – belly, rib cage, upper chest

Exhale – upper chest, rib cage, belly

Repeat several times until there is control over the breathing process. Try not to force the breath – it should be a smooth, wave-like movement. Once this has been achieved, then drop the upper chest breath and just let the breath flow naturally and smoothly as follows:

Inhale – belly, rib cage

Exhale – rib cage, belly

All the stale air will be expelled from the lungs on the exhalation and the inhalation will bring fresh air to all parts of the lungs.

On any given day we take approximately 21,000 breaths, and our lungs remove 400 litres of carbon dioxide from our body.

Shallow breathing confines the gas exchange to the upper part of the lungs, thus inhibiting their cleansing capacity.

The best way to help the lungs do their job of eliminating carbon dioxide and other volatile wastes is to cultivate a habit of deep, diaphragmatic breathing. This pulls air deep into the lungs, fully oxygenating the blood and promoting efficient cleansing.

– Dr Carrie Demers, MD

(Medical Director, Himalayan Institute)

2:1 Breath Ratio – *De-stressing the Body*

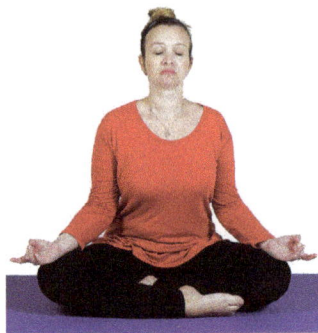

Breathing is part of the autonomic nervous system – it happens whether we are aware of it or not. However, it is one part of the autonomic nervous system that we can override – we can take control of our breathing.

The autonomic nervous system is composed of the parasympathetic nervous system (which helps us 'rest and digest') and the sympathetic nervous system (which engages our 'fight or flight' response). The parasympathetic nervous system decreases the heart rate, lowers the blood pressure and releases muscular tension. The sympathetic nervous system has the opposite affect in that it accelerates our heart rate, raises our blood pressure and tenses our skeletal muscles, all of which are required if we are in a stressful situation that needs to be dealt with.

The problem is that in our very stressful lives it is sometimes difficult to change the 'fight or flight' response to 'rest and digest' and the body stays locked permanently in the stress response.

Through breath control, we can always find our way back to a calm, relaxed breath where the body feels 'safe' and can recuperate and restore.

So the next time you are feeling extremely stressed, notice how you are breathing (in the chest) – your inhalations will be longer than your exhalations. This chest breathing will be increasing your stress levels.

The obvious way to de-stress the body is to increase the exhalation length. In fact, if you make the exhalations twice as long as the inhalations, and keep breathing in this pattern for several minutes, your stress levels, heart rate and blood pressure will drop.

The 2:1 breathing technique is a sure fire way to calm and nurture your nervous system, and the beauty of it is that you can do it anywhere, any time, even while travelling to work on the bus or train or driving the car.

How to practise 2:1 breath ratio

❖ Sit comfortably with the head, neck and spine aligned.

❖ Begin to use the diaphragmatic breath. If it is difficult to unlock the diaphragm, then place a hand on the abdomen and exaggerate the inhalations and exhalations for a few breaths to get things started.

❖ Once the breathing has calmed and you can feel the breath moving the abdomen, then start to count the duration of the inhalations and exhalations and aim to make them equal in length. Most people are comfortable with a 3/3 or 4/4 count. Do this for some time, feeling the body start to relax.

❖ Then start to lengthen the exhalations and allow the inhalations to become a little shorter each time. Gradually adjust the ratio of breath to a ration of 2:1 (e.g., exhaling for 4 and inhaling for 2).

❖ Work on making the transition from one breath to the next a smooth wave-like movement – with no force of any kind.

❖ Do the practice until you feel you have gained control over your breath and are feeling relaxed.

Hand Mudras – *Gestures*

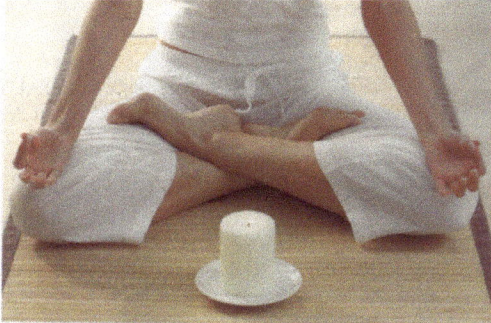

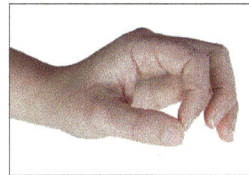
Gyana Mudra

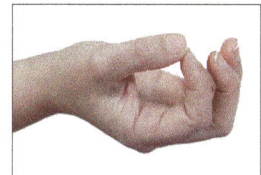
Chin Mudra

In the following pranayama practices, several hand mudras are used. Mudras are an independent branch of yoga, and a study all on their own, so they are not covered here in any great depth. These mudras are used to aid concentration and deepen the awareness.

The two most commonly used mudras in meditation and pranayama practices are Gyana Mudra and Chin Mudra. We lose prana through our hands, and these mudras, which join the thumb and index finger, redirect the prana (energy) back into the body.

Gyana Mudra – *Gesture of Knowledge*

Curl the index fingers into the inside root of the thumbs. The remaining fingers are straight, relaxed and slightly apart. The hands are placed on the knees with the palms facing down.

Chin Mudra – *Gesture of Consciousness*

The same as Gyana Mudra except that the palms of the hands face upwards with the backs of the hands resting on the knees.

Nasagra Mudra – *Nose-tip Position*

The other mudra used in the following pages is Nasagra Mudra. This mudra is used in Nadi Shodhana Pranayama (on following page) to control the flow of breath into alternate nostrils.

Hold the right hand in front of the face. Place the thumb on the right nostril and the index finger and middle finger at the eyebrow centre. The ring finger rests on the left nostril and the little finger curls under and out of the way.

The thumb and the ring finger are used to close off the right and left nostrils alternately to control the flow of breath.

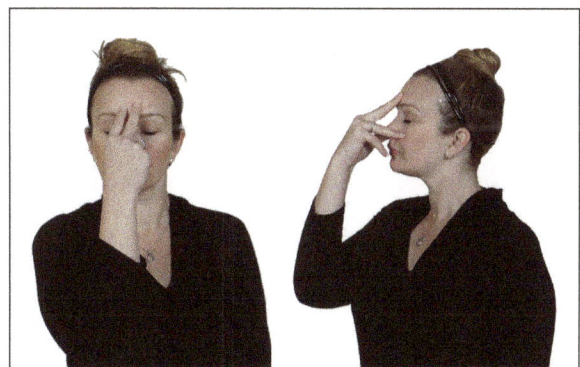
Nasagra Mudra

Nadi Shodhana Pranayama – *Alternate Nostril Breathing*

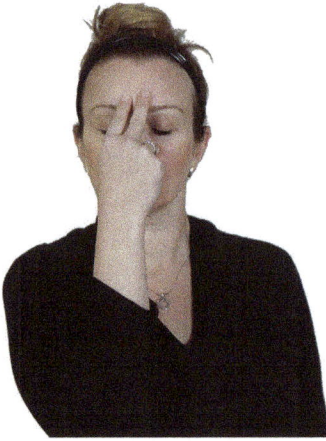

Nadi Shodhana is a balancing pranayama. Its purpose is to balance the flow of breath and energy in the nostrils.

At any given time, either the right or left nostril is flowing more freely and this changes approximately every 90 minutes. There is a cross-over period when both nostrils are open and flowing equally. When we balance this flow of prana, we balance the sympathetic and parasympathetic nervous systems, and the left and right hemispheres of the brain.

In Nadi Shodhana we should aim to keep the breath smooth and subtle and to develop a working relationship with the breath.

Nadi Shodhana is taught in stages and this book will not cover all of them. In the latter stages, breath retention (kumbhaka) and breathing ratios are introduced, but these are best taught by a qualified teacher in a yoga class setting.

Benefits: Nadi Shodhana brings balance to mental and emotional states and benefits the nervous system. It is also an excellent practice to do prior to meditation, as it calms the mind naturally.

Stage 1

Sit in a comfortable meditation position (see page 78) making sure the head and neck are in a straight line with the spine. Close the eyes and relax the whole body. Observe your breath, making sure the diaphragm is not locked and the breathing is relaxed.

Place the right hand in Nasagra Mudra and place the left hand in either Chin or Gyana Mudra (see previous page).

Close the right nostril with the thumb and breathe in through the left nostril for the count of 3 or until the breath ends comfortably. Do not strain.

Close the left nostril with the ring finger while releasing the thumb on the right nostril, and breathe out through the right nostril for the same count. Make sure your inhalations and exhalations are equal.

Then inhale through the right nostril (same count), close off this nostril and breathe out through the left nostril (same count).

This is 1 round; practise up to 10 rounds.

Stage 2

When you have become comfortable with Stage 1, then introduce a ratio of 1:2. For example, if you can breathe in comforably for the count of 4, then exhale for the count of 8. If you breathe in for 5, then exhale for 10.

Keep practising this technique until you are able to manage it with ease.

Note: Further instructions in this practice using breath retention techniques (kumbhaka) should be done with an experienced teacher in a yoga class, however the above (basic) practice will bring balance to your body, mind and nervous system.

The development of Nadi Shodhana should happen over an extended period of time, and each stage should be perfected before moving on to the next.

Bhramari Pranayama –
Humming Bee Breath

Ujjayi Pranayama –
Psychic Breath

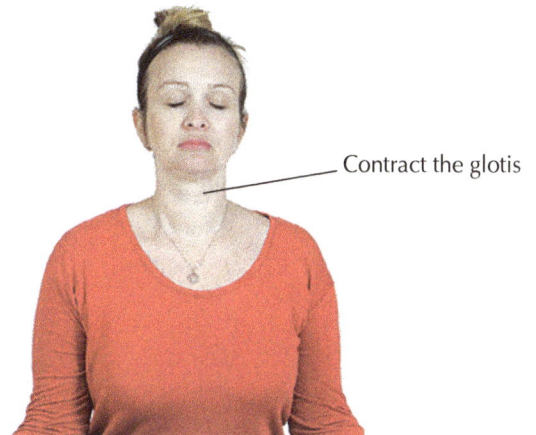

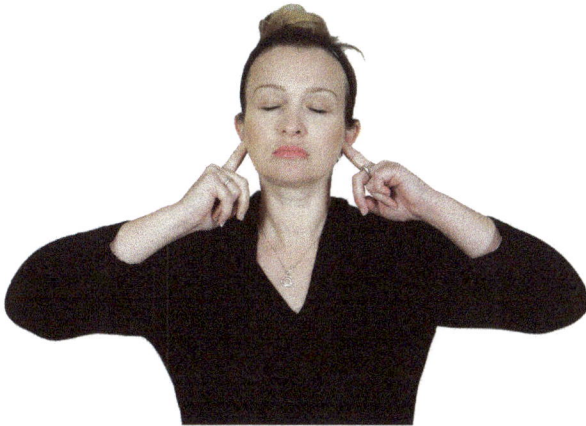

Contract the glotis

Bhramari Pranayama is a tranquillising pranayama which stimulates the parasympathetic nervous system, thereby relaxing the body and drawing the awareness inwards.

Sit comfortably with the spinal cord erect and the head and neck in line with the spine. Close your eyes and relax the whole body.

Relax the jaw with the lips barely touching and the teeth slightly parted. Raise the arms sideways, elbows bent, and use the index fingers to plug the ears (the flaps of the ears may be pressed to avoid placing fingers in the ears).

Bring the awareness to the forehead, breathe in through the nose and exhale slowly while making a steady, controlled humming sound. The sound should be smooth and continuous for the duration of the exhalation. The reverberation should be felt in the front of the skull.

This is 1 round. After exhaling, breath in deeply through the nose and repeat the process.

Benefits: Relieves stress, anxiety and high blood pressure. It can also help to alleviate anger and insomnia. May strengthen the voice.

Ujjayi Pranayama is a tranquillising pranayama which soothes the nervous system and calms the mind.

Sit in a comfortable meditation posture and relax the body. Take your awareness to the breath and stay focused on it until the breath becomes, slow, rhythmic and relaxed.

Then take awareness of the breath to the throat. Focus on the rhythmic and relaxed sound of the breath here.

Now imagine that you are drawing the breath in and out through the throat – not the nostrils. Gently contract the glotis (top of the back of the throat) which slightly hinders the inhalation and exhalation, making the breath longer and deeper and creating a soft sound like the wind in a pipe.

The breath should be long, deep, rhythmic and controlled. Concentrate on the sound made by the breath moving in and out of the throat. This sound should not be so loud that others can hear it, it should only be heard by you, the practitioner.

Benefits: Soothes the nervous system and relieves insomnia. It can also be practised in Shavasana before sleeping. Excellent breathing technique for meditation as it calms the mind very quickly.

Sheetali Pranayama – *Cooling Breath*

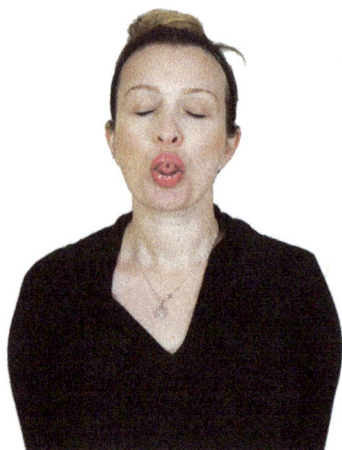

Sheetali Pranayama is a cooling breath and a tranquillising breath. However, about one-third of the population are genetically unable to roll the sides of their tongue into a tube. (In this case you may practise Sheetkari Pranayama instead for similar benefits.)

Sit comfortably, eyes closed with hands in a mudra. Extend the tongue as far as possible and roll the sides of the tongue to form a tube. On inhalation, slowly draw the breath in through the tube, then withdraw the tongue and close the mouth. On exhalation, breathe out slowly through the nose.

The inhalation should make a soft sound, like the wind in the trees, and it should have a cooling effect on the tongue and the roof of the mouth.

This is 1 round; practise 8 rounds to start with and slowly build the number of rounds as you become familiar with this practice.

People with low blood pressure or respiratory disorders should not practise this pranayama.

Benefits: The practice cools the mind as well as the body (especially on hot days). It also helps to physically relax the body as it stimulates the parasympathetic nervous system and has a tranquillising effect on the brain. It may also reduce blood pressure.

Sheetkari Pranayama – *Hissing Breath*

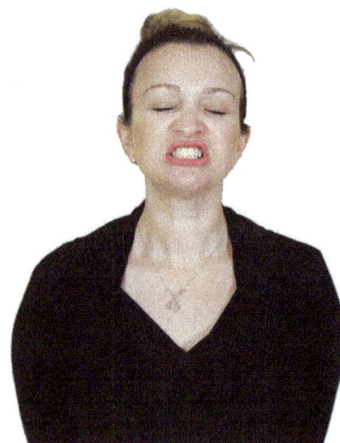

Sheetkari Pranayama is also a cooling breath and a tranquillising breath. This practice may be difficult for people with sensitive teeth.

Sit comfortably, eyes closed with hands in a mudra. Have the teeth barely touching. Part the lips as wide as you can with your teeth and gums fully exposed.

On inhalation, draw the breath in slowly through the teeth, drawing the breath to the back of the throat. At the end of the inhalation, close the lips and breathe out slowly through the nose.

This is 1 round; practice up to 8 rounds to begin with and slowly build the number of rounds as you become familiar with this practice.

Benefits: The practice cools the mind as well as the body (especially on hot days). It also helps to physically relax the body as it stimulates the parasympathetic nervous system and has a tranquillising effect on the brain. It may also reduce blood pressure.

Free Your Breath – Free Your Mind

There are more pranayama practices than have been covered in this book, such as Bhastrika and Kapalbhati, but these techniques are best taught in person by a qualified teacher in a yoga class or ashram setting.

Breathing is the essence of yoga. The breath and the nervous system are closely linked, and when nerves are upset, the breathing is equally affected.

Learning how to witness and observe the breath is probably one of the most powerful practices of all. When we observe the breath we notice that our breathing changes – sometimes it's fast, sometimes slow, it can be deep or shallow, rhythmic or arrhythmic.

Many things affect the way we breathe, such as pleasant or unpleasant emotions, chronic pain (which can restrict our breathing), the sudden intake of breath when we are suddenly shocked, deep sighs when we flop in a chair from exhaustion.

Stress is one of the major contributors to erratic breathing and if we are constantly breathing in a stressful way, it can become a habit which embeds itself permanently into our breathing pattern, resulting in numerous poor health outcomes.

Once we know how to relax our breathing, just being the silent witness, observing the movement of the breath will create a mind/body connection which will in turn calm the nervous system and foster peace of mind.

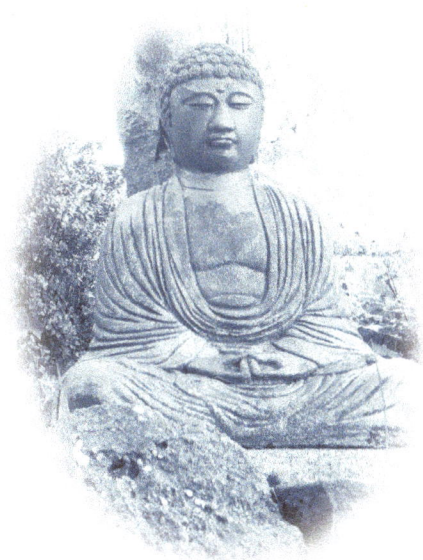

Paying exquisite attention to the breathing in any asana or movement reveals the life of the breath within the body in all its beauty and complexity.

The sensations of renewal and expansion that accompany each inbreath, as well as those of release (and sometimes relief) that are present with each outbreath, become infinitely more vidid.

And these sensations, especially on the outbreath, can be powerfully felt in both body and mind, as built-up tension in particular regions releases and dissolves."

– J Kabat-Zinn, PhD, (Professor of Medicine Emeritus at the University of Massachusetts Medical School)

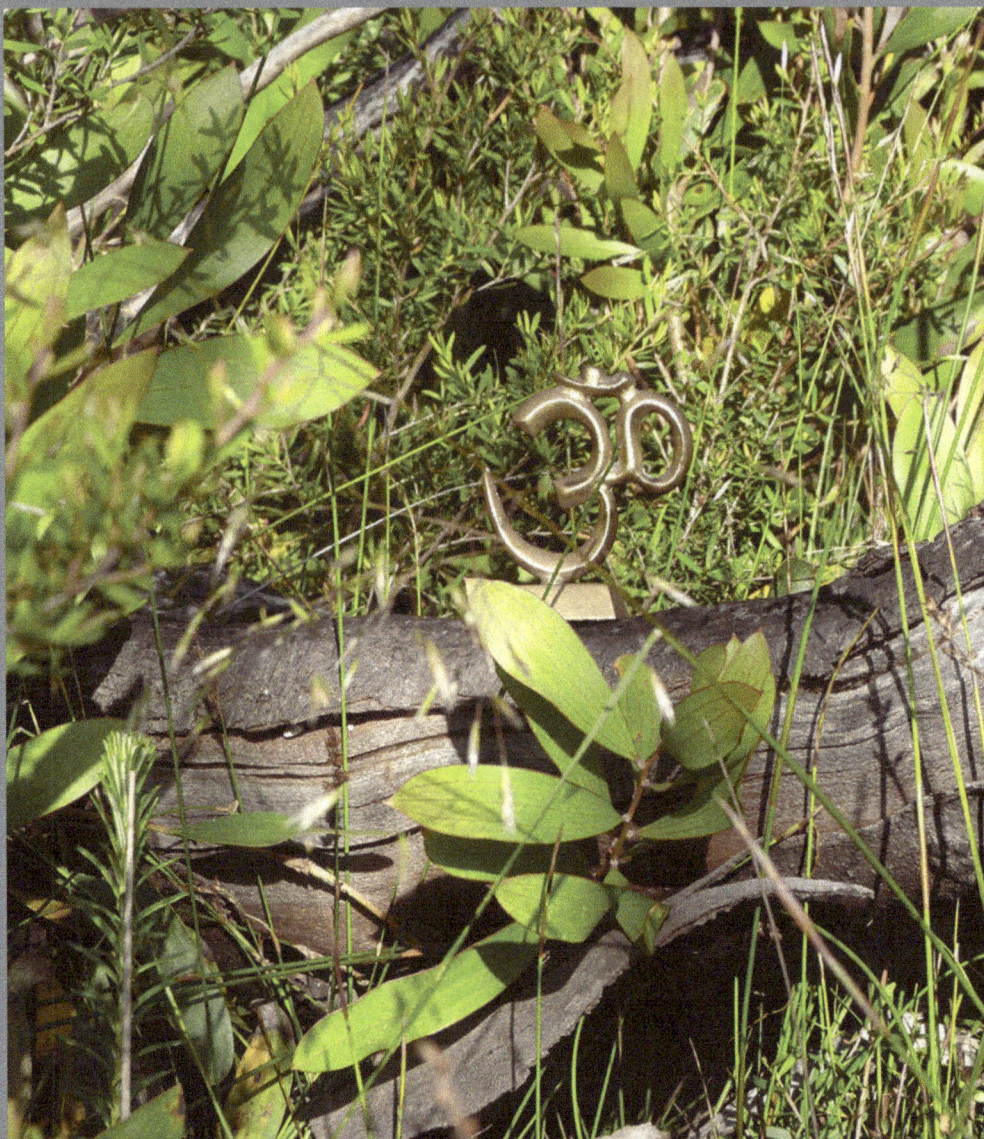

Pratyahara

Relaxation and Sense Withdrawal

Bodies at rest become souls at peace

Relaxation and Sense Withdrawal

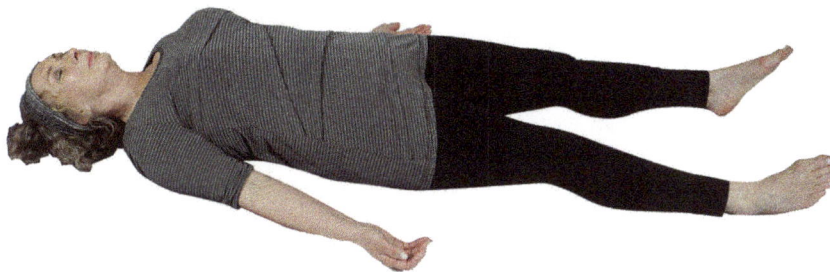

Lying in Shavasana or Corpse Pose is the ideal way to relax the body, mind and spirit. The more practised you become in this pose, the more quickly you can bring total relaxation to the body. Also a lot of healing can take place during this practice, especially if done after asana. It gives the body time to absorb and integrate the physical asana and allows the body to rejuvenate. Shavasana soothes the nerves and reduces fatigue, stress and muscular tension. It can revitalise your entire system.

How to practise relaxation

Lie down on the floor with the feet hip-width apart and the feet falling to the outside which allows the leg muscles to relax and the hips to gently open. Arms are alongside the body, but not touching, palms facing upwards with the fingers lightly curled. Tuck the chin in slightly to lengthen the back of the neck. If you have a sway back or difficulty lying on your back for any length of time, then place a rolled blanket or bolster under your knees.

Imagine your spine is a midline in your body and feel your arms and legs are equidistant from this line. Then start to relax. The body is fully supported by the floor so there is no need to cling to anything. Scan your awareness through the body and if you find any areas of tension or tightness, just imagine you are breathing in and out of these areas and they are gently releasing and letting go.

You can't make relaxation happen but you can work with your breath. Link your awareness with the breath and imagine on each exhalation the body is releasing, relaxing, gently melting down and letting go. Focus on that rhythmical flow of the breath – breathing in what is new, breathing out what is old. Relax as long as you need to.

Come out of Shavasana slowly. Wriggle fingers and toes. Take your time. Then draw the knees to the chest and gently roll to one side. Stay here for a little while, before you use both hands to push yourself up to a sitting position. Sit for a little while and then slowly open your eyes.

Note

Although Shavasana is used during asana sessions to bring balance and relaxation to the body, you don't have to save this amazing practice just for your yoga session. You can do Shavasana any time that we need to revitalise.

The following are a few ideas for a deep and meaningful experience.

❖ You can use an eye pillow if it helps you move more deeply into relaxation.

❖ Place a small cushion under your head.

❖ Use a light blanket if lying in Shavasana for any length of time.

❖ Have some soft music playing in the background.

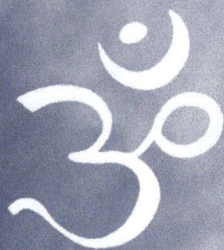

If you look at the sky, what you tend to notice is the objects in it – the passing birds or changing clouds. The ordinary or habitual mind has a tendency to fixate and follow these transient forms without noticing the unchanging and ever present canvas of the sky.

When we bring our attention to rest upon this canvas, we find that it is still, luminous and silent. A mind filled with such awareness has become awakened to its true nature ... We must learn to see the sky and to focus our attention on this unchanging background.

– Donna Farhi
(Yoga Mind, Body & Spirit: A Return to Wholeness)

Dharana and Dhyana

Concentration and Meditation

The Higher Realms of Yoga

Meditation Overview

Yoga, according to Patanjali's Yoga Sutras, is the 'cessation of the fluctuations of the mind.' It is meditation. The ancient yogis and seers only practised asana to enable them to be more flexible so they could sit in meditation longer. So historically, at least, meditation is the heart of yoga.

Many people shy away from this practice as they feel their minds are just too busy and active to be able to settle into meditation. This is the natural state of everyone's mind. The mind has to be trained to meditate. It is like learning a musical instrument or another language – it doesn't happen overnight.

Meditation is not about 'emptying' the mind, it is about being able to concentrate and 'still' the mind. It's about being able to focus and not be distracted by thoughts. Thoughts will still arise in meditation – the idea is to acknowledge them, but not to get into conversation with them.

The ultimate goal in yoga is to become one with the object of meditation: the Self or Universal Consciousness (samadhi). Although this is the goal it is very rare to reach this state. Most serious practitioners achieve a state of high concentration where they are free of the ceaseless chatter that usually accompanies the mind. In meditation, as in all yoga, it is more about the journey rather than the destination. The good news is that we do not have to reach samadhi to reap the benefits of meditation.

The benefits of practising meditation are well documented. Medical studies show that meditation decreases stress levels, and as we already know, stress is the major contributor to most of our illnesses.

There are many ways to approach meditation. The following pages aim to give a simple, straightforward approach to getting started on the amazing journey within.

Look within

How to sit comfortably

In meditation, it is important to be able to sit comfortably for a length of time. If your back and hips feel painful, this will take all of your mind's attention. Being able to sit comfortably removes this obstacle, no matter how flexible or inflexible the body might be.

There is only one rule for sitting comfortably in meditation and that is to sit with the **knees lower than the hips**. This keeps the natural 'S' curve in the spine, puts less pressure on the back and, as a result, the spine feels more supported. There are several ways to do this, depending on your flexibility.

Yoga adepts sit in full Lotus Pose which is out of reach for most people. Swastikasana is far more achievable.

Swastikasana

Sit on the edge of a folded blanket. Start with the legs straight out on the floor. Bend the left leg and place the sole of the foot against the inside of the right thigh. Bend the right leg and place the heel of the foot on the floor in front of the left foot with the sole resting against the left shin. The heels will now be one in front of the other. (Be sure to reverse this position from time to time to keep balance in your seated position). Knees must touch the floor for support. Hands in a Mudra.

Vajrasana

From kneeling, bring the big toes together and separate the heels. Lower the buttocks onto the inside surface of the feet with the heels touching the sides of the hips. Lift and lengthen the spine. The back and head should be in alignment. Place the hands in a mudra.

Blanket stack

It is also possible to stack blankets to a height that ensures your knees will be lower than your hips. If your knees do not reach the floor, then place blankets under the knees. Hands in a mudra.

Meditation stool

Meditation stools are a blessing for inflexible hips. The seat slants forward ensuring the knees are below the hips. Place a blanket under the knees if they feel a bit tender in this position. Hands in a mudra.

The chair

And lastly, if all else fails, use a chair. This is a perfectly valid way to sit in meditation. Make sure that you place a cushion or folded blanket towards the back of the chair so that your knees are lower than your hips. It is also important in this position, to place your feet hip-width apart and have the shins perpendicular to the floor. Hands in a mudra.

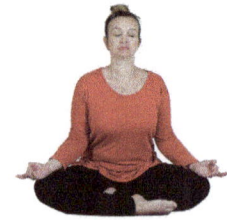

Swastikasana

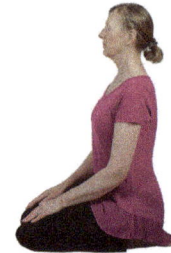

Vajrasana

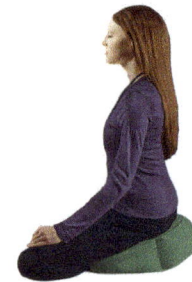

Blanket stack or cushion

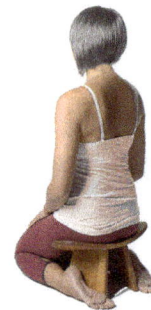

Meditation stool

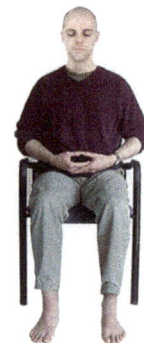

The chair

Gentle Meditation Practices

The following are easy and very gentle meditation practices that may be done by anyone. There are three meditations (and a walking meditation) outlined, but you do not need to practise them in order. Choose one and work with it for a few weeks, then experiment with another. Meditation does not have to be complicated to be effective. A technique is simply a way to anchor and focus the attention. Once you have mastered this, you can allow your awareness to let go into its own peaceful space. This is the ultimate aim of meditation.

Managing discomfort

If you are unable to sit in any of the postures given on the previous page, due to illness, injury or excessive discomfort, then you may opt to lie down in Shavasana. This is also a valid meditation posture, but there is a tendency to lose awareness and fall asleep. So, if possible, sit upright.

If you have a tendency for backache, then you may sit against a wall for support.

Remember that it takes the body time and regular practice to get used to sitting still. It is a training so take it slowly. If you get pins and needles then adjust your position as needed. Also be aware that pins and needles may often be avoided by elevating the buttocks slightly so that there is less pressure on the pelvis. Try sitting on a large cushion and experiment to find what works for you.

Timing

It takes time for the body and mind to settle into a meditative state, due to fluctuating energies and thoughts. Be patient. Give the system time to settle. Start with small challenges, perhaps just 3 minutes to start with, and keep a diary. You will make progress through regularity and consistency. Master these qualities alone and you will soon excel in meditation.

Recording

It is very difficult to guide yourself through meditation initially, because the awareness is untrained. If possible, make a recording on your device of any of the following meditations. Speak slowly and give pauses as needed. Just listening to the sound of your own voice guiding you can be a powerful meditation experience.

Every time you create a gap in the stream of mind, the light of your consciousness grows stronger. One day you may catch yourself smiling at the voice in your head. This means that you no longer take the content of your mind all that seriously, as your sense of self does not depend on it.

– Eckhart Tolle

As gold purified in a furnace loses its impurities and achieves its own true nature, the mind gets rid of the impurities of the attributes of delusion, attachment and purity through meditation and attains Reality.

– Adi Shankara

Stillness Meditation

Adopt a comfortable meditation posture and place your hands in a mudra.

Close your eyes lightly.

Take a deep breath in and slowly exhale, releasing the whole body. . . do this 4 more times . . .

Now start to feel the body becoming still. Start with the toes and feet . . . becoming still. Move up the legs, feel the legs becoming still . . . the buttocks becoming still, the whole back, the shoulders.

Now come to the front of the body. Move your awareness from the pelvis up through the abdomen, the stomach, the chest . . . except for the breath there is no movement . . .

Now come to the fingers, feel the fingers and hands becoming still . . . move your awareness slowly up the arms . . .

Feel the neck becoming still . . . now up into the head and face, feel the forehead becoming still . . . the eyes . . . cheeks, nose, mouth . . . feel the jaws becoming still . . . feel the whole face still, the whole head still . . .

Now feel that the whole body is completely still. It is relaxing into this stillness. Your body is returning to stillness . . .

There may be thoughts, but do not suppress any thoughts – they are just on the periphery of your experience. Do not engage with them, but do not suppress them in any way.

Now let yourself sit for a few moments, just resting in this stillness . . . *(pause for a few moments)*

(Ending) Now, notice your breath . . . notice any sounds around you . . . allow yourself to start making small movements . . . take your time . . . when you are ready, stretch your arms above your head and then stretch any way that you like.

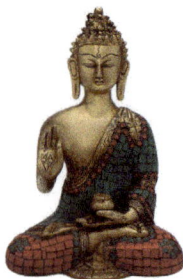

Witnessing Meditation

Adopt a comfortable meditation posture and place your hands in a mudra.

Close your eyes lightly.

Take a deep breath in and slowly exhale, releasing the whole body. . . do this 4 more times . . .

Now become aware of your thoughts, and do not suppress any thoughts. Let yourself think, but at the same time be the witness . . . *(pause for a few moments)*

Thoughts are bubbling up all the time, it is natural, but sometimes you become overwhelmed and stressed by these thoughts. All you have to do is witness, watch, observe these thoughts . . .

After a while they will lose their power, their intensity, because you are stepping back slightly to watch them. Just like watching a movie . . . *(pause for a few moments)*

(Ending) Now, notice your body . . . notice any sounds around you . . . feel your breath . . . allow yourself to start making small movements . . . take your time . . . when you are ready, stretch your arms above your head and then stretch any way that you like.

Relaxing Breath Meditation

This can be short or long, depending on the time you have.

Lie down in Shavasana and close your eyes.

Take a deep breath in and slowly exhale, releasing the whole body. . . do this 4 more times . . .

Now become aware of your breath, the natural flow of the breath . . . do not change it in any way You will start to notice that sometimes your breath is shallow, sometimes deeper and sometimes you might pause in between breaths. This is all natural. Do not change anything . . .

Now feel the breath in the nostrils and just let yourself float in and out with the breath in the nostrils. Let your attention sit lightly on this breath.

Continue for as long as you like . . .

Walking Meditation

One of the most pleasant ways to meditate is to do a walking meditation. In this practice, your awareness is focused totally in the present moment. Very often our thoughts are in the future, thinking about what might happen, or else we are dwelling on the past – something that we are still clinging to from times gone by. What we need to do is to be in the present moment – after all, this is the only time we are really living – not in our past or future.

There is no fixed way to do a walking meditation but the following are the basic principles of the practice. It is so enjoyable that it can easily become part of your daily life.

How to do a walking meditation

This practice is best done in the natural environment as nature has a way of restoring our inner power and is a great source of spiritual nourishment.

Take your time, have no plans for actually getting anywhere and don't take your problems and troubles with you.

Walk mindfully. You can walk with a heel, toe action placing one foot just a little in front of the other, or you can coordinate your breath with your step, inhaling with the right step, exhaling with the left.

You can walk focusing on the movement required to take each step. Notice how the muscles and other body parts coordinate to propel you forward.

If possible, walk with bare feet and really feel grounded and connected to Mother Earth. It is also beneficial to remove glasses or sunglasses (if possible) to let your eyes absorb every aspect of the natural world around you.

Then cycle through your senses one at a time in any order.

❖ Focus on the sense of smell, taking in all the different aromas – especially powerful if walking through the bush.

❖ Let your sense of hearing take over and listen to the sounds of nature all around you. Listen to your footsteps.

❖ When focusing on your sense of touch, reach out and feel the bark of a tree or the soft side of a leaf. Feel the temperature of the air on your skin. Feel the ground underneath your feet.

❖ Our sense of sight is very powerful. Look more closely at everything you see around you: the ants crawling over rocks, the fragile spiderwebs gently swaying in the breeze. And don't forget to look up at the sky and observe the ever-changing cloud formations drifting across the sky.

A feast for all the senses and food for the soul.

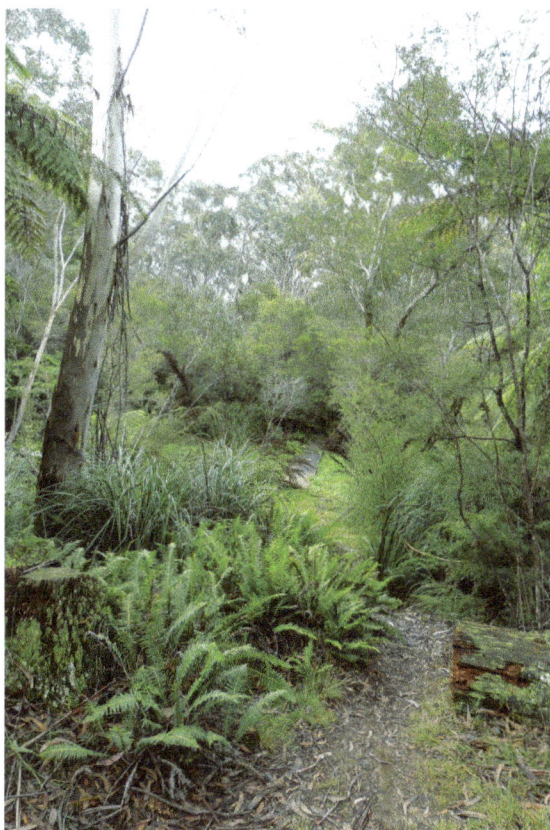

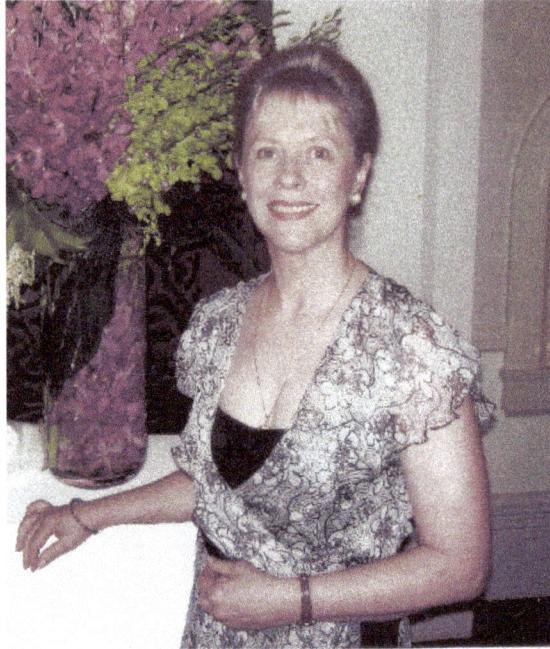

About the Author

Sharon Kirchner lived in Leura, the Blue Mountains, and taught yoga for 16 years in her studio.

Like many yoga teachers, her teaching and personal practice became a hybrid of several yoga disciplines.

Sharon was accredited with the International Yoga Teachers Association, an organisation that encourages their teachers to explore numerous yoga disciplines.

Sharon also completed two years of yoga study at the Satyananda Yoga Academy at Mangrove Mountain. Satyananda Yoga is a multi-faciated and holistic yoga, with an emphasis on the more traditional yoga practices.

In 2002 Sharon attended a three-month Kriya course in Sweden at the Scandinavian Yoga and Meditation School.

In more recent years, Sharon continued her yoga studies through various workshops and was a member of the on-line teaching forum of the Himalayan Institute, Honesdale PA.

www.ingramcontent.com/pod-product-compliance
Lightning Source LLC
Chambersburg PA
CBHW061010030426
42334CB00033B/3438